Sex Positions

3 in 1 Bundle- Climax Enhancing Sex Positions Guided Through Kama Sutra And Tantric Sex Teachings For Sex Life Mastery

Sex Positions

Master The Climax With Advanced Guided Sex Positions For A Better Sex Life, With Pictures

Table Of Contents

Introduction

Thank you for taking the time to download this book: Sex Positions.

This book covers the topic of Sex Positions, and will teach you how to advance your sex life for better and longer lasting sex. This book contains 50+ sexual positions that will drive you wild and leave you begging for more.

At the completion of this book you will have a good understanding of Sex Positions and be able to use and master these positions to reach climax sex.

I hope you find it to be helpful!

Chapter 1: Mastering the Art of Sex

Sex is more than just an expression of animalistic instincts; it is an art. It is an expression of your sexuality and identity. It is also the expression of your love, lust, and affection for your partner.

But, while sex is a primal human need, people are not born with great sex skill. To increase your sexual satisfaction, you must master the art of sex by following these tips:

1. Be confident.
   There's nothing sexier than confidence. Before anyone else can fully love and appreciate your body, you have to love and appreciate your body first. You must believe that you are beautiful and attractive.

2. Pay attention to the foreplay.
   Foreplay is important in increasing your pleasure and improving your overall sexual experience. You must pay attention to foreplay. Make sure to do a lot of torrid kissing, petting, and oral sex before the actual penetration.

3. Practice safe sex.
   You cannot enjoy sex if you are constantly worried about getting pregnant or contracting sexually transmitted disease. To avoid this, it is best to practice safe sex and use condoms and other types of contraception all the time.

4. Try different positions.
   Sex can get boring if you are doing the same sex positions all the time. It is important to try different positions every

now and then. You can find 50+ positions in this book that will totally blow your mind.

5. Act out a fantasy.
   If you want a satisfying sex life, it is important to act out a fantasy. You can organise role-playing games or you can simply act out an erotic movie scene that you and your partner enjoy.

6. Talk dirty to your partner.
   Sometimes, your partner will need some encouragement. It's best to talk dirty. Talking dirty also increases your sexual confidence and empowers you. During intercourse, you can say something sexy like "yes!", "that's so good!", "you're delicious", or "fuck me now".

7. Buy sexy underwear.
   When you have tight, revealing underwear, you'll feel confident and amazing. This confidence will increase your sex performance and the sexual attraction your partner has for you, ultimately heating things up a lot quicker.

8. Let your partner know how desirable he or she is.
   To improve your sexual experience, it's a good idea to let your partner know how desirable he/she is. This will improve the connection and enhance the overall quality of sexual intercourse. You can say something like "you're hot babe" or "you're a sex god".

9. Maintain eye contact with your partner during sex.
   Maintaining eye contact with your partner allows you to establish a deep connection with him/her and it also improves the overall sexual experience.

10. Use props.

Props add excitement and pleasure. It's best to use props such as blindfolds, feathers, handcuffs, whips and even food.

11. Wear costumes.

Costumes are visually appealing. They also add a lot of excitement and novelty into your lovemaking. Maybe she can be the Cop and he can be the one in 'trouble'.

12. Make love in public places.

Having sex in public places is not only exciting. It also has an element of danger that increases pleasure. You do not have to do it in a park or in a public toilet. You can do it in your car or against an open hotel window.

13. Make love in different parts of your house.

If having sex in public places is too much for you, you can have sex in the different parts of your house instead. You can have sex on your couch, on the piano, on the kitchen counter, and even on the stairs.

14. Pay attention to your partner's erogenous zones.

To have better sex, it is important to pay attention to the erogenous zones of your partner.

If you're a woman, you need to pay attention to the penis during foreplay. All men love a good blowjob. When you are giving your man oral pleasure, try to do it slowly and let yourself linger. Take the penis, one centimetre at a time. You can suck and lick, using the lipstick strategy – brush the head of the penis against your lips as if you are applying a lipstick. It is also important to pay attention to your partner's other erogenous zones such as the ears, neck, frenulum, and nipples.

If you're a man, you need to pay attention to the woman's clitoris. This part of her vagina has over eight thousand nerve endings. You can play with her clitoris using your fingers or your tongue. It is also best to pay attention to her other erogenous zones such as the ears, neck, nipples, feet, and even her scalp.

15. Keep a little bit of clothes on during sex.
    There's something a little exciting and kinky about keeping a little bit of your clothes on during intercourse. Keep them on until your partner rips them off.

16. Make loud noises during intercourse.
    Try to let go of all your inhibitions. When you're having sex with your partner, it is important to make loud noises during sex. The kind that would keep all your neighbours awake. Using the positions and techniques in this book, you wont have any other option but to scream. So get used to it.

17. Be playful.
    Sex is not something that you should take seriously. To have an amazing and deeply satisfying sex life, be playful, have a laugh and get comfortable with each other. Pillow fights or a playful wrestling fight during foreplay can cure the awkwardness and set the sexual confidence to wear it should be.

18. Eat foods that increase sexual performance.

If you want to increase your sexual performance and drive, you should tweak your diet and add foods that increase libido and stamina such as cucumber, kale, flaxseed oil, pine nuts, garlic, broccoli, blueberries, blackberries, avocados, oysters, almonds, strawberries, seafood, arugula, figs, and citrus. You can also eat a lot of meat, red wine, pumpkin seeds, fatty fish, dark chocolate, and strawberries.

19. Watch porn with your partner.
    Women actually like porn too, but not the ones that focus on the pounding or the genitals. To improve the sexual experience, it would be a good idea to watch porn with your partner.

20. Make a little home movie.
    Recording your sexual intercourse will motivate you and your partner to take sex to the next level. If you want wild sex, it's a good idea to record a little homemade porn. See what it's like and make a better and longer one each time.

Sex is one of the basic primal needs of human beings. It is also good exercise, providing stress relief and strengthening your immune system. Most of all, it is an expression of love and maybe lust, making it one of the most beautiful things about being human and one of the most pleasurable things that you should enjoy.

Chapter 2: Easy Sex Positions

If you're a beginner just starting out towards your sex life journey then these positions are for you requiring low flexibility, energy, and skill. Here are the best sex positions for beginners:

Sex Position #1 Missionary Position

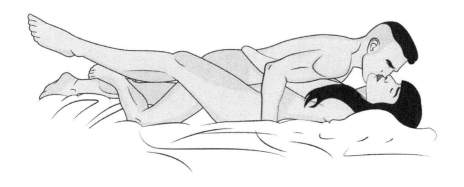

The missionary position is one of the most basic sex positions. It is also the most commonly used. This sex position is intimate and it creates a more romantic atmosphere allowing both the man and the woman to maintain an eye contact while making love. They could also kiss and express affection for each other.

Most women love the intimacy that comes with the classic missionary position, which is why it's a good position to start with. Holding eye contact and kissing each others ears and neck will get things heated really quick, making it comfortable for both partners to change things up with more confident based positions.

How To Do It

The woman has to lie on her back with her legs spread wide and the man should climb on top of her front on. This is one of the easiest positions for the man to access the Vagina.

How to Make This Position Hotter

1. Make sure that the woman orgasms before the intercourse. It's no secret that women do not get orgasms from intercourse alone. To make sex more pleasurable for her, it is important that she orgasms before the actual intercourse. The man should do a little fingering or give her oral pleasure before penetration. This strategy makes missionary sex more enjoyable and pleasurable for both partners.

2. The man should not do all the work. The woman should also move her hips in a wavelike undulating pattern.

3. Get rough! Try to scratch your partner's back or bite his/her shoulder blades. This would definitely turn your partner on.

4. Whisper something in your lover's ear. You can whisper sweet things or you can whisper naughty things.

5. Breathe more. The more you breathe, the more body sensations you feel. This will help you feel more pleasure.

Sex Position #2 CAT or Coital Alignment Technique

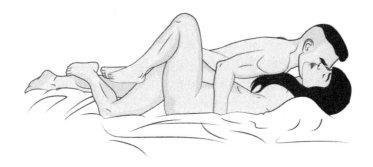

The coital alignment technique or CAT is a variation of the missionary position. It's also known as grinding the core. This sex position was created to maximize clitoral stimulation. An American psychotherapist named Edward Eichel in 1998 first defined it.

How To Do It

The man lies above the woman, but moves upward so his erection would point down instead of pointing up. This means that the dorsal side of the penis is pressing against the clitoris. This increases clitoral stimulation and helps the woman experience more pleasure during sex and ultimately achieve orgasm.

The woman can also wrap her legs around the man's waist to deepen the penetration. She should also keep her hips tilted up during the intercourse so the clitoris is stimulated with precision.

To achieve better sexual experience using the coital alignment technique, the man should make sure that his weight is evenly distributed. He should rest part of his weight on the woman's chest.

How to Make This Position Hotter

To make sex more pleasurable, the man should also move in more than one direction. He should move in a sensual and slow rocking motion and not in the usual thrusting motion. It is best to vary the pace, rhythm and angle of the thrusts as targeting different areas in different speeds causes more pleasure for the woman. The extra tips from the previous missionary position can be used also.

Sex Position #3 Woman On Top

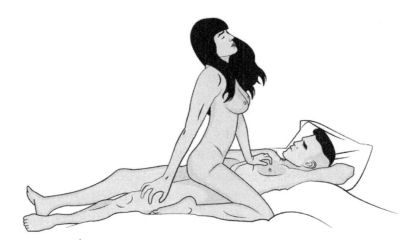

Woman on top or cowgirl position is one of the most common and easiest sex positions. It is enjoyable for both parties and it helps the woman feel in control and empowered. This position also allows the man to freely move his hands around the woman's breasts and other parts of her body. It also gives the man a great view of the woman's body and movement, which is immensely satisfying.

How To Do It

The man has to lie on his back and the woman straddles across his pelvis facing forward. The woman could either kneel or squat. She will then align her vagina with the man's penis and lower herself to allow the man to penetrate her.

This position allows the woman to control the rhythm, the pace, and the extent of vaginal penetration. The man can freely touch the woman's breasts, buttocks, or clitoris while the woman moves "up and down" in a circular motion.

This position is best during pregnancy because the weight of the man is not on the woman. Men like this position because it allows them to have a full frontal view of the woman.

How to Make This Position Hotter

Turning the lights on for this position is ideal, as it will increase the sexual attraction the man had for the woman. This Position puts the woman in full control so talking dirty to your partner will definitely heat things up which will then cause the man to prove himself in the position after when he is then doing the work.

Sex Position #4 Modified Girl On Top

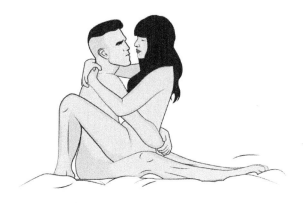

This position also allows the woman to control the movement during intercourse just like the CAT but creates deeper and more forceful thrusts. This is also more intimate than the classic girl on top position, allowing more hugging, kissing, and other expressions of attention.

How To Do It

The man must lie on the floor/bed laying his back against a wall and the woman should climb on top of him. But, instead of sitting upright on top of her man, she should lean down against his chest, placing her hand on either side of his head. This will make her more secure when moving, creating more control. If the woman is strong in the arms and legs, she can also lean back with her hands on the bed and bounce on her partner while he rests for the next position.

This position provides maximum clitoral stimulation and it can be pleasurable for the man, too. To maximize pleasure, the man must also thrust forward and move his hips up while the woman is moving in the "up and down" or circular motion.

How to Make This Position Hotter

Making out with each other, while the man grabs the buttocks and breasts can increase the sexual tension. This position also has easy access towards kissing, licking, biting and sucking the neck and ears.

Sex Position #5 The Doggie Style

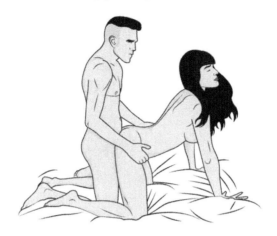

Doggie style is one of the most popular sex positions, especially for men because of its animalistic vibe. It is exciting for both men and women especially due to its wild take, making it an amazing visual treat for men and a good position to try during pregnancy.

How to Do It

The woman must be on all fours. The man kneels behind her and enters.

The doggy style is a versatile position that can help the sex partner move in whatever way they like. It encourages breast stimulation and it helps the woman feel uninhibited because the man cannot see her face. It's easier for her to let go allowing her to comfortably moan, grunt, and talk dirty as much as she wants.

The doggy style is a rough sex position that many people enjoy. It also provides awesome G-spot stimulation. To increase the force and orgasm, the man can place one leg up, similar to a lunge position.

How to Make This Position Hotter

The woman and man can dirty talk to each other while the man can also spank her on the buttocks if his partner desires. If the woman turns her head and looks at her partner this also increases the sexual connection for the man due to eye contact at a high status.

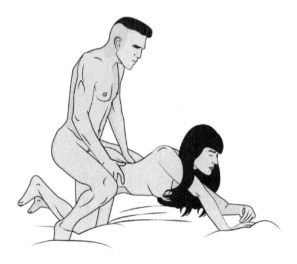

Extra Tip: If you have strong legs, going two legged, in a squat position or in a lunge position with one knee down and one up, can be even more advanced and climax efficient.

Sex Position #6 Spooning

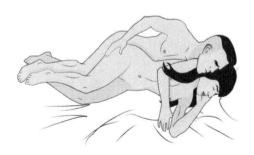

Spooning is one of the most intimate sex positions. It allows the man to cuddle his partner while they are having intercourse. This position releases the love hormone called oxytocin, which brightens the mood. Having intercourse in this position can actually makes you feel happier.

This position combines the "body to body" closeness of intimate and romantic sex positions and the excitement of rear entry. This position provides superior G-spot penetration and clitoral stimulation, allowing both the man and the woman to have access to the different hotspots of the woman's body. This is also a good position to try anal sex.

How to Do It

The woman should lie on her side with the man behind her, facing the same direction. To find the right angle for entry, the woman may have to lift her top leg or lean forward. Then, the man enters from behind. The man can grope the woman's breasts or play with her clitoris during intercourse.

How to Make It Hotter

To make this position even hotter, the woman can bend her knee to create a triangle. This will allow her to accommodate her man better. It also gives her more leverage to move and match his thrusts. If the woman is flexible and a little acrobatic, she can hold her leg up. Then, she can grab her partner's butt to intensify the penetration and thrust. This trick can make the intercourse more memorable, exciting, and wild.

Sex Position #7 The Tight Squeeze

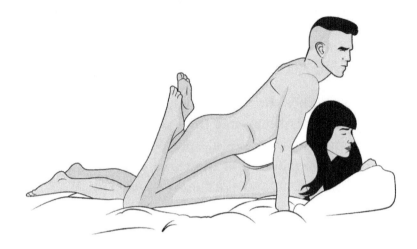

This is an intimate rear entry position that's incredibly easy to do. It creates intimate and feel-good friction. Allowing the man to easily kiss the woman's lips or neck during intercourse.

How to Do It

The woman should lie down on her stomach, keeping her legs straight or crossed. She can rest her arms on her side or she can stretch them out in front of her. The man will then stretch his body over her, resting his elbows or hands on the bed so he doesn't put his entire body weight on his partner. The man will then position his legs beyond the woman's legs and enters her. Placing a pillow under the woman allows a better angle for the man to easily slide in and out from and hit the G-spot.

How to Make This Position Hotter

To enjoy the full benefit of this position, the woman should rock her buttocks back and forth while he's thrusting. This will increase the impact of the thrusts and the pleasure.

Sex Position #8 The Cowboy

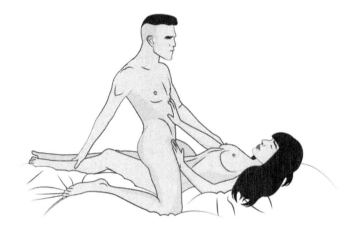

The cowboy is a romantic position that gives the man dominance. It is relatively easy to do and it does not require a lot of energy. The man can also put on an actual cowboy hat just for fun.

How to Do It

The woman should lie back and the man should climb on top and straddle her. He then needs to insert his penis through the tight opening. The tightness increases the pleasure and intensity of the penetration, which is good for both the man and the woman.

How Make This Position Hotter

The man can fondle the woman's breasts or he can tie/handcuff her to the bedpost for added excitement and pleasure.

Sex Position #9 The Drill

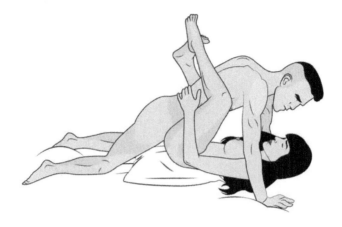

The drill is similar to the missionary position. This position provides superior G-spot stimulation, which is easy to perform, providing maximum pleasure.

How to Do It

The woman must lie on her back and the man should climb on top of her. As he enters her, she should wrap her legs around the guy's waist. The raised leg adds intimacy to the position and improves the penetration angle.

How Make This Position Hotter

Having a pillow underneath the woman's lower back makes it easier for the man to enter and hit the G-spot. The couple can kiss each other and more importantly the man can kiss and bite the woman's breasts and neck during intercourse.

Sex Position #10 Sixty Nine

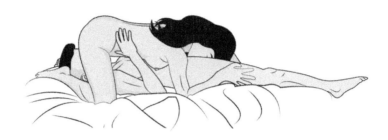

The 69 is one of the easiest and dirtiest sex positions used in foreplay. You can also do this in between different sex positions. This position is pleasurable for both partners, but it gives the woman more oral pleasure.

How to Do It

The man should be lying underneath the woman. The vagina should be in the guy's face and the woman's face should be on the man's penis. This is the classic version of the 69. You can also reverse this position.

How to Make This Position Hotter

To get the most out of this position, the man can use his hands to stimulate the woman's clitoris and the G-spot. To enjoy this position, you must let yourself go and enjoy the moment.

It is also important to keep the woman wet, so she can truly enjoy the experience. It's best to use different kinds of lubricants such as lick-able lubricants, flavored lubricants, and warming lubricants. The man should also focus on giving the woman a G-spot massage.

If the woman is flexible, she can bend over backwards instead of directly facing the penis. Of course, the woman must do a lot of yoga to be able to do this.

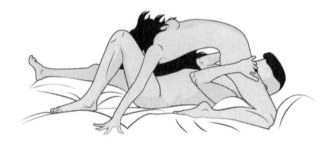

Chapter 3: Intermediate Sex Positions

These positions are best for slightly fitter people with moderate sex skills and flexibility. The positions also require moderate stamina and energy, making them more exciting and satisfying. If you're looking for a new position to try, it may be a good idea to try these positions.

Sex Position #11 Butterfly

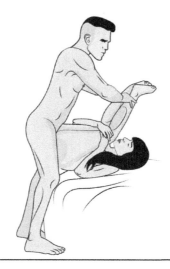

The butterfly sex position allows deep penetration. This position is visually satisfying for the man and it provides the woman great clitoral stimulation, making it wild and exciting.

How to Do It

The woman should lie at the edge of a table or a bed, with the man standing in front of her. The man should lift the woman's hips upwards and place her legs on his shoulders or hold them with his hands. If this is too difficult, the woman can simply place her legs on the man's hips.

How to Make This Position Hotter

The man can give the woman oral pleasure before transitioning to this position. He can also kiss and bite her inner legs or squeeze her breast during intercourse.

Putting a cushion underneath the woman's butt is also a good idea. This way, the man won't get too tired of holding up her legs.

Sex Position #12 Time Bomb

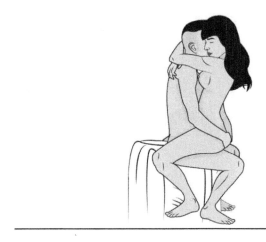

This sex position is intimate, with the girl on top. The time bomb allows you to kiss your partner and maintain eye contact during intercourse. The man can touch or kiss the woman's breast and neck during sex.

This position provides maximum G-spot and clitoris stimulation and it also gives the woman a strong sense of control.

How To Do It

The man should sit on a chair and then the woman should climb on top, facing him. The man should place his hands on her buttocks for support as she rocks up and down.

How To Make This Hotter

To make this hotter, the woman can lean back and allow the man to suck her breasts or kiss her neck. This position is perfect for wild sex, but to get the most out of this, it's a good idea to vary the speed and the rhythm of the lovemaking.

This Position is a great one to do in the back seat of a car also.

<u>Sex Position #13 Face to Face</u>

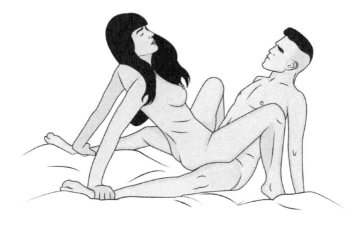

This position is perfect for slow and relaxing sex. It is intimate and it allows the couple to look into each other's eyes and kiss, making it one of the most sensual sex positions ever recorded in the Kama sutra.

How to Do It

The couple should sit opposite each other. Then, the woman must slide into his lap and sit on top of him. The man should put his feet together to provide some kind of cradle for his partner. Then, the woman can place the penis inside her and start to rock up and down.

How to Make This Position Hotter

To make this position hotter, the woman can lean back and allow the man to have a better view of her jiggling breasts.

Sex Position #14 The Right Angle

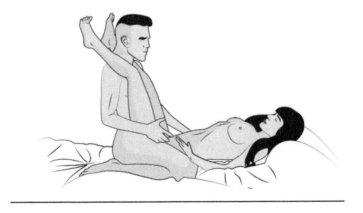

The right angle is a bit similar to the butterfly. This position helps increase the penetration by increasing the depth forced in. This position is not intimate but it is wild.

How to Do It

The woman should lie down in the right angle position, with feet up. Then, the man sits down on the bed with his legs open and stretched out. He can grab the woman's legs and rest them on his shoulders. The man can also place his hands on the woman's butt or waist and lift her up and down. This allows deep penetration.

How to Make This Position Hotter

To get the best from this position, the couple should maintain eye contact. This will increase the intimacy and enhance the sexual experience. The man can also occasionally kiss the woman's legs or grope her breasts.

This position is versatile. You can do this in the bedroom and even in a hallway.

Sex Position #15 Standing Up

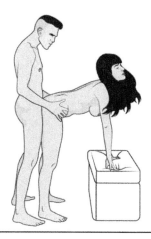

This position is great for hitting the G-spot. It also creates deep penetration allowing the man to have a good view of his partner's butt.

How to Do It

The woman should turn and face away from her partner. Once positioned the woman must bend over placing her hands on the wall or her knees for leverage. The man should stand behind her, also having his hands placed on her hips or butt to pull her closer with each thrust.

How to Make This Position Hotter

To make this position wilder, the man can use a clitoral vibrator to enhance her pleasure and increase her chances of orgasm. If your partner is into it, he can slap her buttocks for increased sexual tension. He can also rub or kiss her back during intercourse.

Sex Position #16 Reverse Cowgirl

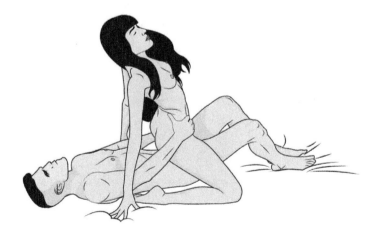

This position makes the woman feel empowered, giving the man the amazing view of his partner's butt, stimulating her G-spot at the same time.

How to Do It

The man should lie on his back with the woman sitting on top of him, facing his feet. She could also squat over him with her feet on the bed. When the woman is well lubricated, she should hold the base of the guy's penis and slowly lower herself onto him. She then has to start moving up and down. She can maintain her balance by placing her hands in front of her or on the guy's thigh.

How to Make This Position Hotter

To make this position hotter, the man can place his hands on the woman's waist and help her move up and down. He can also squeeze and slap her butt during intercourse or kiss her back.

Sex Position #17 The Padlock

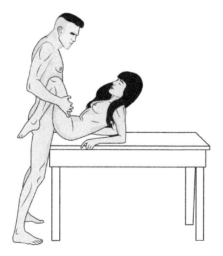

If you want to make love in the office or in the laundry room, this is the perfect position for you. This position allows both the man and the woman to control the rhythm of lovemaking. It also gives the man more access to the woman's body.

How to Do It

The woman can sit on a washing machine, office table, or countertop. The man must stand in front of her with the woman wrapping her legs around his waist. He can grab her butt or suck her breasts during intercourse.

How to Make This Position Hotter

This is an easy position to do in the kitchen or maybe even on the bathroom sink in a public toilet. Making eye contact and talking dirty will definitely heat things up just that little bit more.

Sex Position #18 The Kneeling Lotus

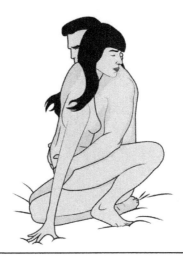

The kneeling lotus creates better movement between the genitals, allowing the couple to move in a fluid rocking motion. This position provides an optimal angle for penetration, while providing great G-spot stimulation. The man has free access to the woman's breasts during intercourse and the woman has a strong feeling of power and dominance. This position is great for people with average weight, low flexibility, and moderate energy.

How to Do It

To get into this position, the man must kneel back and the woman sits onto his lap, facing him. She should then wrap her legs around her partner and wrap her arms around him for support. The couple can whisper sweet nothings or do dirty talk while in this position.

How to Make This Position Hotter

This position is very intimate, so making eye contact and kissing/biting the neck and ears will increase the sexual tension.

Sex Position #19 Kneeling Mastery Position

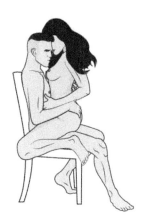

This position is something that all lovers of varying skill level and fitness can do. It is erotic, intimate, and it gives the couple a lot of opportunity to kiss, fondle, and caress each other.

How To Do It

The man should sit on a sofa or chair and the woman should straddle him, facing him. The man can place his hands on his partner's buttocks to help her move up and down.

How to Make This Position Hotter

Pulling her hair and talking dirty is a perfect combination to use in this position. Making sure you are very close to each other will increase the clitoral stimulation, therefor making it easier for you and your partner to have an orgasm.

Sex Position #20 The Lotus

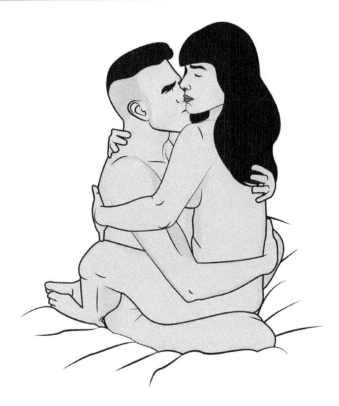

This is a sensual Tantric position that's recorded in the ancient book of love. This awesome sex position is perfect for yoga fanatics. It allows you to sync your breathing and movement for an intimate and romantic position that couples of varying fitness and skill level can try.

How to Do It

The man should get into the traditional lotus position. If this is too difficult, he can simply cross his legs. The woman then climbs on top of him and sits on his lap. She should then wrap her legs around his waist as he can then penetrate her.

How to Make This Position Hotter

The couple should embrace each other during intercourse and kiss with shared breath. The woman should exhale and her man inhales and vice versa. She must rock her pelvis as she inhales, tightening her vaginal muscles.

Sex Position #21 Leapfrog

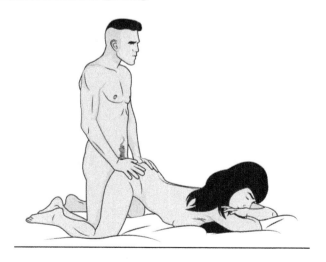

The leapfrog is a variation of the doggy style. This position promotes female orgasm as it provides superior clitoral and G-spot stimulation.

How To Do It

The woman should start on all fours, with the man kneeling behind her like in the doggy position. As he enters her, she should lower herself down and rest her weight on her forearms.

How To Make This Position Hotter

To make this position hotter, the man can stimulate the woman's clitoris during intercourse using his fingers. He can also kiss her back and squeeze her buttocks and maybe even slap it.

Sex Position #22 The Ballerina

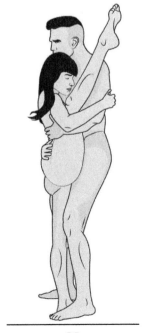

The ballerina is a complicated position and recommended only for women with yoga-like flexibility. This Tantric position is both intimate and wild.

How to Do It

The couple should stand facing each other. Then, the woman should lift one foot and rest it on the man's shoulder. If she cannot do this, she can simply hook her foot around her guy's waist.

How to Make This Position Hotter

To get the best out of this position, it's best to kiss your partner while you are having intercourse. This could improve the experience and increase pleasure. Lifting your partner and pushing her up against the wall while you thrust will also spice things up that little bit more.

Sex Position #23 Teaspoons Sex Position

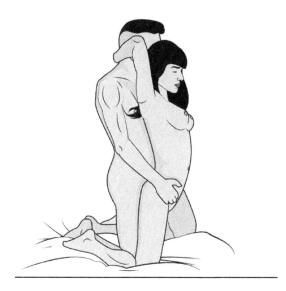

This is a rear entry position that's incredibly intimate and romantic. It has the connectivity of spooning and intensity of the doggy style.

How to Do It

The woman should kneel and the man should also kneel behind her and penetrate her. If you encounter difficulty in aligning the genitals, it's best to use a pillow or cushion.

How to Make This Position Hotter

The man can play with the woman's clitoris or breasts during intercourse. He can also kiss her lips, neck, and shoulders to increase the tension.

<u>Sex Position #24 Victory</u>

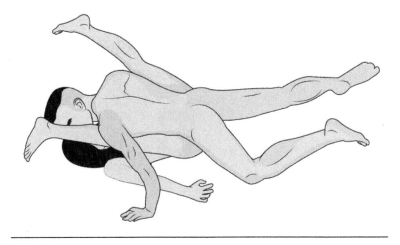

Victory is a daring variation of the missionary position, making it hot and perfect for women who are not too shy.

How to Do It

The woman should lie on her back with the man on top of her, as the man enters her, she needs to extend her legs out to the ceiling in a V-shape position.

This amazing sex position creates maximum penetration and G-spot stimulation. Allowing the man to kiss the woman's legs or fondle her breasts during sex.

How to Make This Position Hotter

Tying or handcuffing your partner's hand to the bed will definitely heat things up with this position. Investing in some rope or fake handcuffs could make a huge difference if you want to take your sex life to that next level.

Sex Position #25 Bended Knee

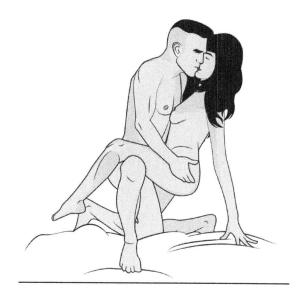

This face-to-face position is intimate and fun to do. It allows the couple to kiss and grope each other during sex.

How To Do It

The man and the woman should kneel facing each other, with the woman raising one leg over the man's opposite thigh. The man enters her and places his hands on her waist for support.

How to Make This Position Hotter

The man can rub the women's clitoris for extra stimulation while holding eye contact at the same time. The man can also use his knee to help with thrusting his woman up and down faster.

Sex Position #26 Lap Dance

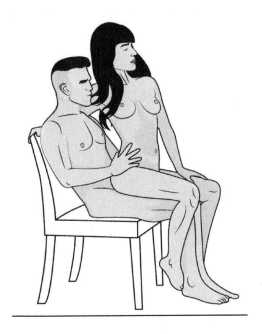

This is one of the highest rated sex positions because of its level of pleasure. It is a versatile sex position that you can do on the sofa, on the bed, on a stool or on a chair.

How to Do It

The man should sit on a sofa or a chair and then the woman sits on his lap, facing away.

How To Make This Position Hotter

To make this position more intense, the woman can do circular thrusting motion instead of the usual "up and down" thrusts while playing with her clitoris during intercourse. The man can pull her hair if she's into that also.

Chapter 4: Advanced Sex Positions

If you want to experience extreme, crazy and exciting positions, these are the ones you should pursue. Although these sex positions are challenging and require maximum flexibility, they will make you beg for more and add some extra spiciness into your sex life. Here's a list of some of the complicated and unconventional sex positions that you should try at least once in your life.

Sex Position #27 Folded Desk Chair

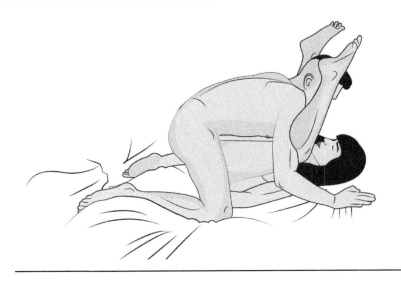

This sex position is intimate and requires great flexibility on the part of the woman. It is great for romance and it stimulates the G-spot. This position deepens the penetration so it is perfect for guys with a smaller penis.

How To Do It

The woman should raise her legs up towards her face in a folded desk chair position and the man should kneel in front of her, pushing her legs down with his shoulders and enter her.

How to Make This Hotter

To make this position hotter, the woman can raise her legs as high as she can. The man can also occasionally kiss her legs and vary the speed and rhythm of the lovemaking.

Sex Position #28 Stand And Carry

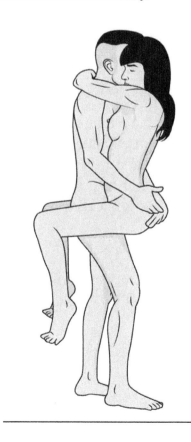

This position is hot because of the intimacy and strength it creates. It's also romantic and allows the couple to kiss and whisper sweet nothings to each other during sex.

This sex position is not for the faint of heart and this is only great for physically fit people. The woman must also be petite or thin, so it's easier for the man to carry her.

How To Do It

The man should stand and then carry the woman up by holding her buttocks. The woman then wraps her legs around her partner's waist and places her arms around him.

How To Make It Hotter

To make this position wilder and more pleasurable, the man can kiss the woman's breasts or lips.

This position can strain the man's back or neck so it's important to do this for no more than two minutes. It is also best to do this against the wall so the man can last longer and is able to thrust with more force. If you want take things even further, doing this position in a public toilet or a dark alley is as easy option if you're into that.

Sex Position #29 The Dolphin

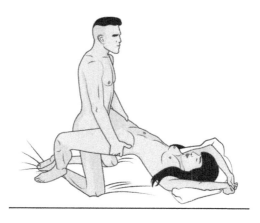

The dolphin is a yoga-like sex position that provides great G-spot stimulation. The woman's head is inverted during sex, which means that the blood flow to her brain is increased, this improving the level of pleasure, excitement, and sensations that she feels during sex. This position requires moderate to high flexibility on the part of the woman.

How To Do It

The woman should lie on her back and then slowly raise her back, abdomen, and knees from the bed into a bridge position. The man then kneels on top of her, holds her waist, and then enters her.

How To Make This Position Hotter

To take this position to the next level, the man can lift the woman's hips higher. He can also fondle her breasts during sex.

This sex position is challenging and you shouldn't hold this for too long as the increased blood flow to the head could lead to dizziness and blackouts.

Sex Position #30 Wheel Barrow

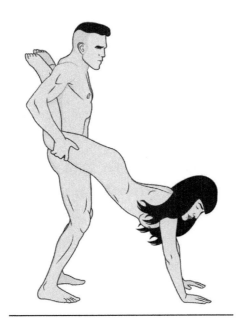

This position provides equal gender dominance, creating great G-spot stimulation and requiring high energy. This is definitely one of the most difficult, exciting, and crazier sex positions. You should try this at least once in your life.

How To Do It

The woman should be in the plank position with the hands and feet on the floor with her legs slightly apart. Her partner stands behind her and grabs her legs up and penetrates her. The woman can match the man's thrusts by moving forward and backward.

The woman needs to have yoga-like strength to be able to carry her weight. She can also hold the weight on her elbows and wrap her legs around the man's waist for additional support.

How To Make This Position Hotter

If the woman is strong enough to hold herself up with her legs wrapped around her partner and the man can hold the rest of the weight with one hand, he can use his other hand to rub his partners clitoris or slap his woman's buttocks for extra pleasure. Talking dirty in this position is also a great idea due to the power and rarity of this position.

Sex Position #31 Deep Impact

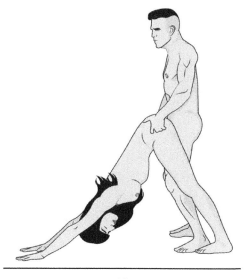

Deep impact provides deep penetration and can be pleasurable for both the man and woman. It is great for passionate and rough sex, including either vaginal or anal sex.

How To Do It

The woman should straighten her legs and create a triangle like shape by supporting herself evenly with her hands and feet. The man should then stand behind her and access the vagina with his penis and begin thrusting.

How To Make This Position Hotter

He can hold up her buttocks to deepen the penetration and spank her while thrusting. This position is great for deep penetration especially if you have a smaller penis and want to penetrate from behind.

Sex Position #32 Sybian

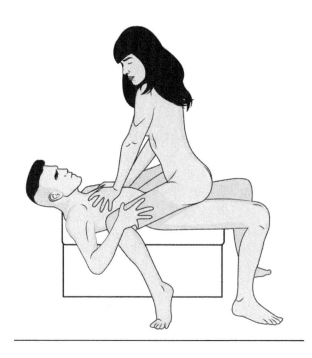

This wild position would leave you crying out for more, requiring strength and flexibility on the part of the man.

How To Do It

To get into this position, the man must lie on his back and then lift his knees, belly, back, chest, and head from the stool or bed. The woman climbs on top of him and guides his penis inside her.

This position is incredibly hard to do. To make it easier, the man can sit on a stool and then slowly bend his back and bring his head and arms down so both his feet and arms touch the ground. The woman will then climb on top of him and straddle him.

How To Make This Position Hotter

This position is very powerful for the woman so it's a perfect opportunity for the woman to talk dirty to her partner. Holding eye contact will also stimulate increased sexual tension.

Sex Position #33 The Triumph Arc

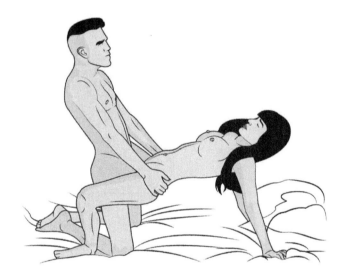

The triumph arch is a romantic sex position that provides great G-spot stimulation. But, it also requires a high level of flexibility on the woman's part. This is one of the most challenging sex positions. In fact, its difficulty rating is 10/10.

How To Do It

The man should kneel on the bed between the woman's legs. The woman must lift her buttocks up from the bed and form an arc shape. This requires core strength from the woman.

How To Make This Position Hotter

Rubbing the clitoris and talking dirty is also a perfect way to making this position more interesting

Sex Position #34 The Plow

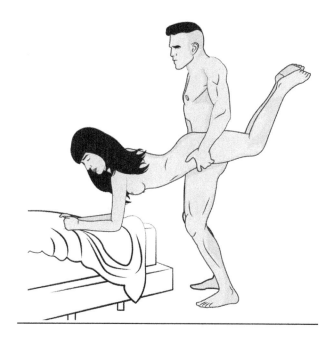

The plow is one of the most difficult and challenging sex positions. It is best for fit and athletic couples. This wild position provides excellent G-spot stimulation, because the woman's body is angled downward so it's easier for the penis to stimulate that part of the vagina. This position is also good for couples that are trying to have a baby.

How To Do It

The woman should lie on the edge of the bed facing down. She should support herself with her elbows and then the man steps between her legs and lifts up her hips, penetrating her from behind.

How To Make This Position Hotter

As this position is quite similar to the wheelbarrow, the man can hold the weight of his partner with one hand using his other hand to rub his partners clitoris or slap his woman's buttocks for extra pleasure. Talking dirty in this position is also a great idea due to the power and rarity of this position.

Sex Position #35 The Suspended Scissors

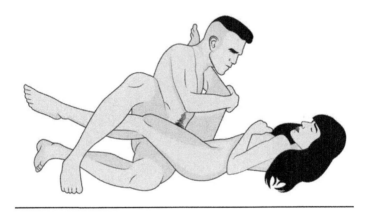

This sex position is not only difficult it is also outrageous. But, if you want to spice up your sex life and add excitement to your lovemaking, you should definitely try this.

This position requires high levels of strength and flexibility for both partners. The suspended scissors is definitely hard-core.

How To Do It

The man should stand still and hold the woman's waist for support. Then she should put one hand on the floor and the other hand on her partner's arm. She should place her legs by the sides of the man. One of her legs must intersect with her partner's leg.

This position increases the blood flow to the woman's head so it increases her pleasure and excitement.

How To Make This Position Hotter

Handcuffing or tying your partners hands to the bed will definitely make things more interesting for this position as it gives the man more power, increasing the sexual tension for the woman.

Sex Position #36 The London Bridge

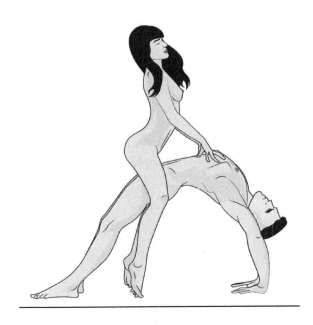

The London Bridge is a complicated sex position that can be performed by athletic and yogic couple. This position is wild, exciting, and incredibly difficult.

How to Do It

The man should lie on his back with his arms above his head, palms down. Then, while taking a deep breath, he should lift his knees, back, and head from the ground and into the yoga wheel pose. The woman then climbs on top of her and guide's his penis into her vagina.

This position is extremely pleasurable for the man because it increases the blood flow to his brain. It is also extremely enjoyable and exciting.

How To Make This Position Hotter

This position is very powerful for the woman so it's a perfect opportunity for the woman to talk dirty to her partner.

Sex Position #37 The G-Force

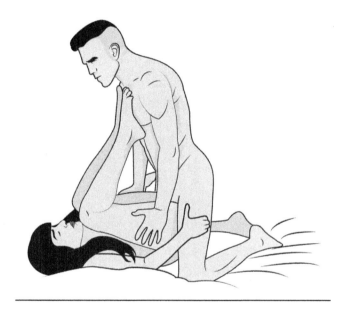

This is a daring and challenging position that provides great G-force stimulation. It's also great for both vaginal and anal sex.

How To Do It

The woman should lie on her back and pull her knees towards her chest. The man should kneel in front of her and grab her feet with his hands, while the man thrusts forward to penetrate her. To increase the level of pleasure, the woman should place her feet on her mans chest, with the man placing his hands on his partner's hips. This will give him extra power and control.

How To Make This Position Hotter

Handcuffing or tying your partner's hands to the bed and maybe even blindfolding her will increase the sexual tension especially if dirty talk is involved also. Squeezing and rubbing your partner's buttocks and thighs will also induce extra pleasure for the woman.

Sex Position #38 The Butter Churner

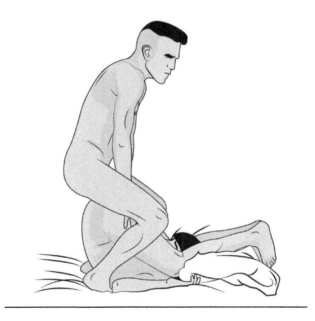

The butter churner is an intimate sex position that's best for men and woman with flexibility and strength. This provides deep penetration and superior G-spot stimulation.

How To Do It

The woman should lie down on her back and flip her legs and knees towards her chest. The man then needs to squat above her, holding her legs and entering from the top.

How To Make This Position Hotter

This position is dirty and is more about focusing on hitting the G-Spot. The couple can talk dirty to each other and create an emotional connection by looking deeply at each other's eyes.

Sex Position #39 The Burning Man

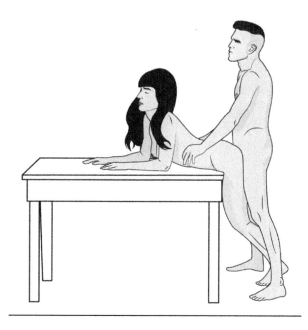

The burning man is one of the hottest rear entry sex positions. It is great for both anal and vaginal sex. This position tightens the vagina and improves the intensity of the penetration. A perfect position to do in the kitchen.

How to Do It

The woman faces the countertop and then slowly rests her upper body on it. The man enters from behind.

How To Make This Position Hotter

Slapping your partner's buttocks and thrusting fiercely against the bench is a good way to make this position hotter. The man can also lean over and grope his partner's breast during thrusts.

Sex Position #40 Swiss Ball Blitz

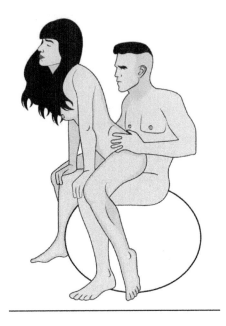

This sex positions requires an Exercise Ball allowing for faster and stronger penetrations. It can easily make a woman Orgasm once the right rhythm is mastered.

How to Do It

The man first sits on the ball as he would on a chair and the woman then sits on him entering the penis from behind. Once comfortable and stable, the man will then need to hold his partners waste and begin pushing him self directly up and down through his legs. It might be a good idea to place the exercise ball close to a bed or wall so if you do fall off balance, you have something to keep you up.

How To Make This Position Hotter

Mastering the rhythm is a huge skill that you will need to master, making it easier for your partner to orgasm. Maybe you can set up a foreplay situation where the man or woman is the personal trainer and the other is the client. This will definitely induce more sexual tension, as you can also talk dirty in terms of being the trainer or client also.

Sex Position #41 Waterfall

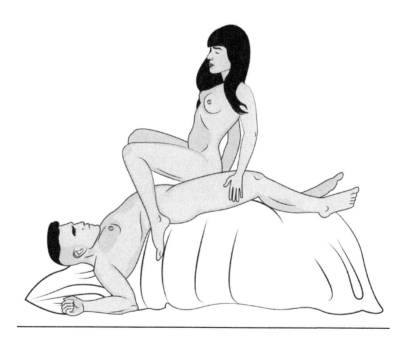

This position doesn't require much strength and is easily done on a bed. For once the man will experience a head rush but this will create a higher sexual experience for him in doing so.

How to Do It

In this position the man will need to lay his backside on the bed with his shoulders resting on the floor. The woman can then squat or sit on the man frontally pushing her self up and down directly.

How To Make This Position Hotter

The woman can switch between facing towards her man or away. The reverse position of this would give her man a great angle of the woman's buttocks jiggling up and down during thrusts.

Sex Position #42 Snow Angel

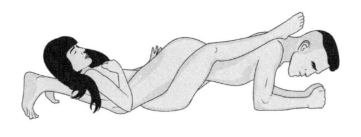

This position will hit a spot the woman most likely hasn't experienced before and who knows maybe it might be the one to make her reach climax the quickest. This position is mainly for the woman because the man cannot see her partner but it's something different and something that will definitely make things exciting.

How to Do It

The woman will need to lie on her back with her legs spread out. After she is comfortable the man will need to come over the top of her and lay on his stomach with his elbows on the floor between her legs. The woman can then hold his butt pushing the man up and pulling him down, while also thrusting her self.

How To Make This Position Hotter

The woman can rub her hands along her mans inner thighs and hamstrings as this is a very sensitive area for men, creating extra sexual pleasure.

Sex Position #43 Seated Wheelbarrow

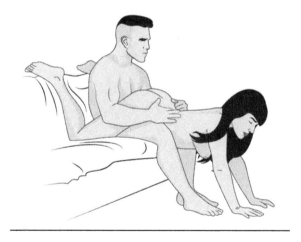

The Seated Wheelbarrow is an easier version compared the standing wheelbarrow, especially for the man. To make this positions easier the woman can but a bench or chair in front of her and rest her elbows on there instead.

How to Do It

In this position the man will need to sit down on the edge of a bed. Once done, the woman can lie on the floor in front of him with her legs spread, the man can then grab her legs and put them in-between his waist. He will need to thrust using his legs.

How To Make This Position Hotter

The man can lean back and put his hands on the bed to acquire more strength by being able to use both his arms and legs to create a more powerful thrust. He can also slap or fondle with his partners buttocks.

Sex Position #44 Crucifixion

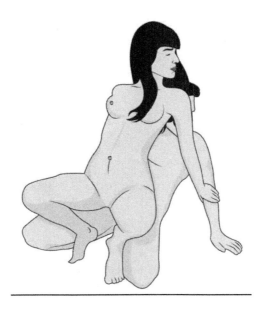

The crucifixion is an advanced sex position, which targets the G-spot. The woman must have strong legs and arms to hold her self up in this squatting position where as the man can rest in this on.

How to Do It

The man must sit on his knees then lean back holding himself up with his arms. Once in this position the woman can put her feet in-between her partner's legs and squat down sliding into the penis.

How To Make This Position Hotter

In this position the man can lick and kiss his partner's back and neck. Talking dirty is recommended also.

Sex Position #45 Torch

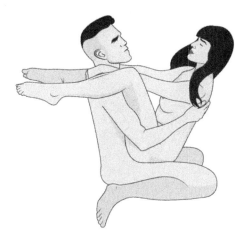

The Torch position is actually easier than it looks but is still for advanced couples. This one is powerful and intimate at the same time due to the eye contact that is made.

How to Do It

The man must kneel on his knees like he started out in the previous position, once comfortable, the woman needs to rest her legs on top of her mans shoulders laying her back on the bed. Once this is done the man must insert his penis into his partners vagina and then lift his partner upright holding her back towards him.

How To Make This Position Hotter

Making strong eye contact and kissing each other will spice things up in the position. The woman can also use her arms to pull her closer towards her partner to create deeper thrusts.

Sex Position #46 Reverse Plank

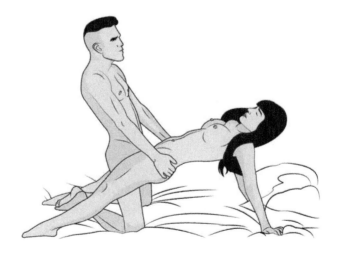

The Reverse Plank is like the wheelbarrow but the man doesn't have to use as much energy holding most of the weight. This

Position is great for both partners as it puts the man in power and gives him a great view of his partner's breasts from above.

How to Do It

The woman must lay legs spread, with her back up right supporting herself upright with her arms. The man needs to kneel in-between her legs and lift her buttocks up with his hands. Once done the man will need to insert his penis into her vagina.

How To Make This Position Hotter

Squeezing your partner's buttocks while you talk dirty to her is the best way to make this position hotter.

<u>Sex Position #47 The Lock</u>

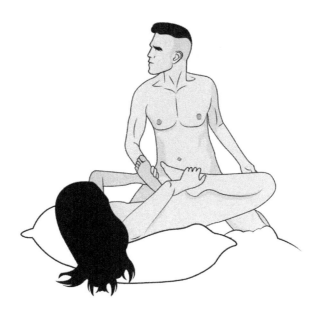

61

The lock is something for the adventurous couples that like the role of being dominant or submissive. This hits a different spot of the vagina making it very pleasurable for the woman.

How to Do It

The woman will need to lay on her stomach bending her legs and heels towards her buttocks, once done she will then need to reach behind and grab her feet. Her partner can help by leading and stretching her arms and legs. It is also important to lie a thick pillow down before this, as it allows the man to get a better angle of penetration. Once the woman is sorted, the man will need to kneel down and insert his penis inside of the vagina.

How To Make This Position Hotter

The man can use handcuffs or rope to tie everything together. Not only does this make things a lot hotter but also it's easier for the woman. Talking dirty and maybe even pulling her hair could also turn you partner on that little bit more.

Sex Position #48 Screw Driver

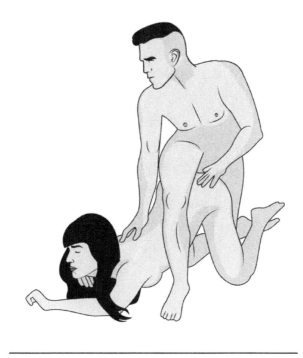

This position is a more advanced position of the doggy style. It allows deeper penetrations, ultimately making it more pleasurable for the woman.

How to Do It

The woman needs to be on all fours with her arms lying across the bed. The man will then need to kneel and place his strongest leg over the woman and then insert his penis inside the woman.

How To Make This Position Hotter

The man can reach below and play with his partners clitoris at the same time as thrusting and in-between he can also slap and fondle with the woman's buttocks. Even some dirty talk while 'riding' your partner will make this position more intense.

Sex Position #49 Mermaid

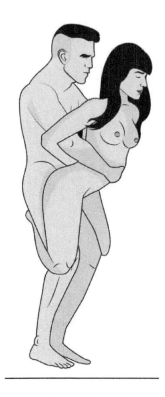

The mermaid position requires a lot of strength especially on the woman's side. This is a very unique and powerful position if you can master it's definitely something you should try once you are super advanced in bed.

How to Do It

Both partners need to stand upright with the woman facing away from her partner in front of him. She must then put her hands behind her back so her partner has room to put his arms through and pick the woman up. Once done the woman will then need to position her legs wrapped around her partner's upper legs so the man can then guide his penis into the vagina. This position requires teamwork, so work together in trying to make this as comfortable as possible.

How To Make This Position Hotter

Ways to make things more interesting could be handcuffing your woman's hands together to make it easier and at the same time boosting the sexual tension. Planning a foreplay... Maybe your partner is your dance instructor and the role-play leads to this position.

Sex Position #50 T-Bone

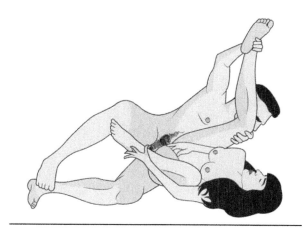

The T-Bone is a unique sex position that is actually quite rare. This position targets the G-Spot perfectly, making it perfect for climax sex.

How to Do It

Both couples need to lie down on the floor, bed or even kitchen table. The woman will need to pull her knees towards her face, however she will need to open them out and wide, opening up her vagina for easy access. Once sorted the man will need to lie across forming a T shape, he can then guide his penis into his partner's vagina.

How To Make This Position Hotter

The man can bite and kiss his partner's leg and also with one hand rub her clitoris. At the same time as this, he can also talk to dirty to his partner.

Sex Position #51 Advanced Leap Frog

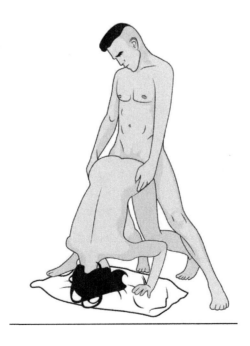

This is a great position to do on a harder surface. Most women love doggy style, and this one takes it to a new level, making it even more exciting. Men also love this as it gives a perfect view of their partner's buttocks.

How to Do It

Just like doggy style, the woman will need to be on all fours, however she will need to be planted on the palms of her feet and hands (Like a leap frog). Once in this position the man will need to bend his knees slightly and insert his penis into the vagina.

How To Make This Position Hotter

Talking dirty and slapping your partner's buttocks in this position will definitely spice things up. If you're more adventurous you can also use a whip, if that kind of thing turns both of you on.

Sex Position #52 Rabbit Ears

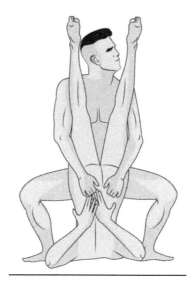

This is a great advanced sex position that is definitely one you should try. Due to the woman being upside down, this will cause the blood flow to fall down causing increased sensations and a head rush. This hits a different zone of the vagina and who knows ,maybe this might be where your partners G-Spot is.

How to Do It

Firstly the woman will need lie down on her back, lifting her legs up in the air. Her partner will then need to grab and lift her legs directly upwards so she is resting on her head and shoulders. Leaning against a wall can make things easier also. Once the woman is upright and comfortable the man will then need to squat upright and enter her from the front. The man will need to control the thrusts here.

How To Make This Position Hotter

He can spank and grab his partner's buttocks and also bite and lick her legs and feet... if you're into that. This isn't a position a woman can hold for a long amount of time so making sure your thrusts are deeper and faster for her to reach orgasm is recommended.

Sex Position #54 The Plank

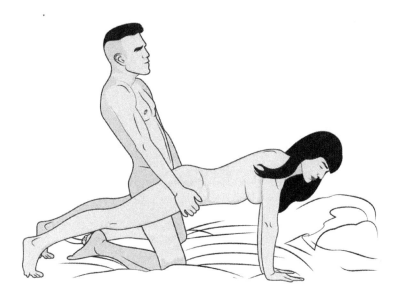

This position is for strong women who can hold a plank comfortably. It is a perfect angle for thrusting and makes it easy for the man to penetrate into the vagina while on his knees.

How to Do It

The woman will need to start off in a plank position, holding herself up with her elbows or preferably her hands, with her legs spread apart enough for her partner to kneel in between. The man will then kneel or squat in between her legs and enter the vagina from behind.

How To Make This Position Hotter

Rubbing the clitoris while thrusting can increase the sensation for the woman and increase the chances of creating an orgasm.

Pulling her hair in this position will also spice things up if you're willing to take a dirtier approach.

Sex Position #55 Half Split's

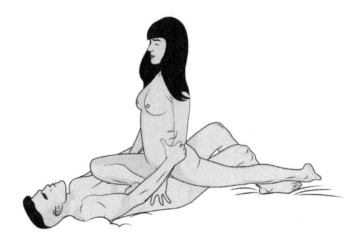

In this Sex position at first it seems quite hard but once you get the hang of it you will really enjoy it and it's actually quite easy for the women to thrust her self up and down. The man doesn't need to do much work here.

How to Do It

The man will lie down on his back normally, making it as easy as possible for his partner to sit on top of him while she positions her self to do the splits. The woman can bend the leg in front of her to allow a wide range of motion when thrusting. She can also spread her legs out in a more comfortable position that isn't too hard to stretch out to. You'll be surprised that you can actually do this position even if you're not that flexible.

How To Make This Position Hotter

The man can play with her breasts and make eye contacts while talking dirty. This position could also be easily set up as a Gymnast instructor teaches student scenario. Planning your positions around a foreplay idea like this always turns the heat up that little bit more.

Chapter 5: Tantric Sex Tips

We are living in a stressful world that trained us to do things fast. We are constantly running out of time. No wonder that quickies are becoming more popular.

Tantra is the art of practicing conscious and romantic sex in order to develop authentic love and passionate connection.

Here are some tantric tips that you can practice to improve your sex life:

1. Engage in a tantric skill
When you kiss your partner, you should try to share your partner's breath. This will make the kiss more intimate. To do this, you need to inhale when your partner exhales and vice versa. This practice will allow you to immerse in the sensations of intimacy and closeness.

2. Give your partner a tantric massage
The tantric massage is sensual and it improves the blood circulation throughout the body. It helps you fight stress and curb impulses, preventing premature ejaculation and helps older men to achieve orgasm.

To do this:
- Rub some massage oil on your hands and then start to massage your partner's lower back in a circular motion. Then, move your hands up to the neck. Repeat this process at least six times.
- Massage your partner's back as if you are kneading a pizza.
- Turn your partner over. Slowly caress your partner's feet using the kneading stroke. Then gently rotate each toe at least six times.

- Massage your partner's hands, neck, shoulders, and breasts.
- If you're a woman, give your partner a lingam massage. Massage your mans penis by squeezing its shaft and moving your hands upward as if you're "milking" it. Go up and down and then make circles. It is also important to stimulate the male G-spot, which is located between his balls and anus.

3. Turn your bedroom into a sex sanctuary

To improve your overall sexual experience, it's a good idea to turn your bedroom into a sex sanctuary. Keep it clean and clutter free and make sure you have new sheets every week. You can also spray exotic and sexy scents around your bedroom to increase your libido and sexual performance.

4. Use aromatherapy

Aromatherapy has been used for many years to cure different medical conditions. It can also help increase passion, libido, and sexual intensity. If you want to improve your sex life then it's a good idea to diffuse the following essential oils in your bedroom:

- Rose – This is a romantic oil that increases your sexual confidence and self-esteem. It also increases semen production and circulation.
- Ylang- ylang – This oil has a sweet and exotic scent and it is a natural aphrodisiac.
- Sandalwood – This is one of the oldest and most popular perfume materials. It is a tension reliever and it boosts your libido.
- Neroli – This essential oil is used as an aphrodisiac in many countries. It improves confidence and reduces feelings of anger.
- Jasmine – This essential oil has a sweet smell and strong aphrodisiac qualities.
- Cinnamon – This essential oil increases your stamina

and energy. If you want to increase your sexual stamina and add spice into your relationship, you should try this.

Remember that sex is not a mere act. It is an expression of love and affection. If you want to improve your connection with your partner, it would be a good idea to try the ancient tantric techniques.

Chapter 6: Exercises to Improve Libido, Sexual Stamina, Flexibility, and Performance

Some of the sex positions contained in this book are complicated and challenging. To perform these positions optimally, follow the list of exercises here:

1. Tongue Push-ups
This may seem funny, but your jaw or tongue could cramp up during oral sex. To prevent this, you can do tongue pushups by pushing the tip of your tongue into the front roof of your mouth. Doing this at least 10 times a day can increase your tongue stamina during oral sex.

2. Pranayama or Breathing Exercises
Pranayama is a breathing exercise that can help relax your body and increase the circulation of your energy. To do this, do ten rounds of breathing through your right nostril. Use your finger or thumb to cover your left nostril. Then, cover your right nostril, and take 10 breaths using only your left nostril.

3. Do abs and lower back exercises
Your core muscles and lower back muscles are used in almost every sex position. To increase your stamina and flexibility, it's good to try lower back and abs exercises. Try pushups, planks, squats, and deadlifts.

4. Try yoga
Yoga is essential when practicing Tantric sex. Yoga increases your strength and flexibility. It also increases your sexual stamina and confidence. To improve your sexual performance, you should try the following yoga poses:

1.   Pigeon pose

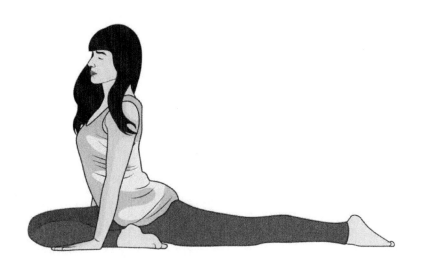

2.   Eagle pose

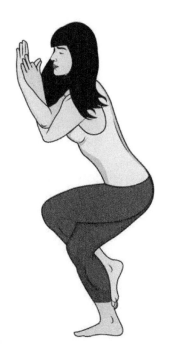

3.   Bridge pose

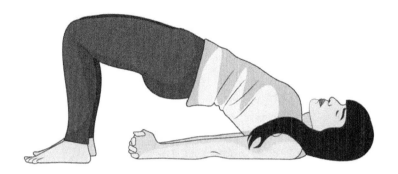

4.   Downward Dog

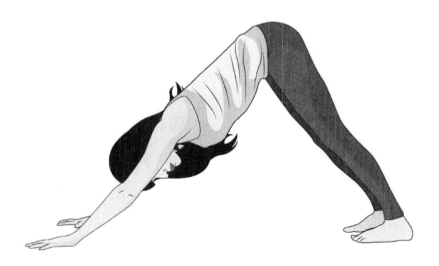

5. Cobra Pose

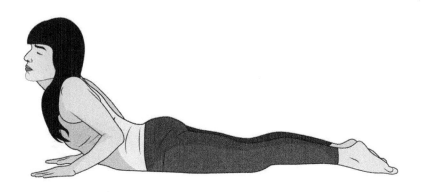

6.   Plank

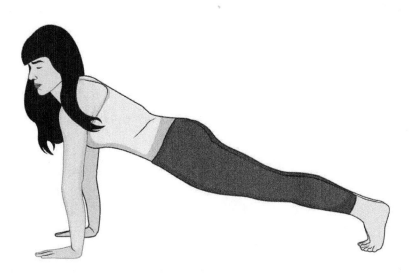

7.   Bound angle pose

These physical exercises don't just increase your flexibility and stamina; they also improve your confidence, which is essential in improving your sexual performance.

Moving from Basic to Advanced Sex Positions

It is recommended that you begin with the basic sex positions first. That includes missionary, woman on top, and doggie positions. These are the easiest positions to try and they are also the most comfortable. When you get the hang of those positions, move to intermediate positions such as butterfly, time bomb, face to face, the right angle, and the lovelock. They require a bit more flexibility.

In the mean time you should try the exercises mentioned here in this chapter. They will help you improve your strength and flexibility. Once you feel more fit and conditioned, you can try one of the advanced sex positions mentioned in this book.

Do the easier ones first like folded chair, and deep impact. They are positions where one partner can lend a helping hand and provide support while maintaining the position. Reserve tougher positions like wheelbarrow and others for later.

Tips on How to Last Longer in Bed

Sex won't be that much fun if the deed is done in two minutes. So, how do you last longer? Here are a few tips:

1. Tongue Back Push
Run your tongue's tip around the roof of your mouth while keeping your mouth closed. Doing this while you're having sex will take your mind off thinking about ejaculating.

2. The Snooze Button
Consider this as an instant way to stop you from ejaculating. In case you went for it too far and you're nearing the point of no return, then try this technique. There is this area in between your anus and your balls.

When you begin to climax, press on this point. Remember to hold it down as if your life depended on it. You will feel contractions down there but keep holding until you have put your ejaculation to a complete halt. Doing this will distract you from focusing too much on your genitals and thus cooling you down; making you last longer.

3. Switch Your Focus
Sometimes all you have to do is to stop focusing on the sensations you are getting. You will feel the muscles in your legs and buttocks tighten, as you get closer to your peak. Maybe try to just look into the eyes of your partner instead of her body.

At this point, slow down. Go into a slow in and out motion and relax your muscles. Look at your partner and focus on her reactions to what you are doing. Keep that satisfied look on her face in your view.

4. Breathe
Once you feel aroused and nearing climax, start breathing deep. Breathe slowly. One of the reasons why you can't last that long is that you rush and take really short breaths. Deep breathing using the full power of your diaphragm relaxes your muscles – especially the ones that matter down there. Take a deep breath, hold for 3 seconds and then exhale. Repeat the steps until you are relaxed and ready for another round. Eventually you last longer.

5. Stamina Kegels

Do regular kegel exercises but this time focus on releasing the tension in your PC muscle (the muscle between your testicles and anus). The goal here is not to build strength but to gain better control. Try flexing your PC muscle alone without any tension from the other tissues in the area. Practice 5 minutes each day until you develop the right muscle memory. Soon you will be able to release the tension in your PC muscle on demand. Doing 3 sets of 20 Reps for 2 seconds each time is a great way to start. Following this every day and slowly increasing the reps and sets will strengthen your PC muscle and allow you to have longer lasting sex.

Conclusion

Thanks again for taking the time to purchase this book!

You should now have a good understanding of Sex Positions, and be able to use these positions and skills to advance and master your sex life.

If you enjoyed this book, please take the time to leave me a review on Amazon. I appreciate your honest feedback, and it really helps me to continue producing high quality books.

KAMA SUTRA

Master The Art Of Love Making Through Advanced Kama Sutra Orgasm Stimulating Sex Positions Guide, With Pictures

Table of Contents

Introduction

Congratulations on purchasing the book, **Kama Sutra: Master The Art Of Love Through Kama Sutra Sex Positions**. For centuries, the ancient Indian Hindi text of the Kama Sutra has been synonymous with discussions on sexual intercourse and the art of lovemaking. The full text in itself is quite lengthy and often tedious to read. In fact, Kama Sutra discusses more topics about human relationships beyond sexual intercourse, but it is the content revolving around human sexuality that has captured the attention of Kama Sutra enthusiasts for millennia.

Are you looking for techniques to enhance your sexual prowess, give more pleasure and satisfaction to your partner, or reinvigorate your sexual relationship or compatibility? In this book, you will find a concise, easy-to-read guide based on the texts of the Kama Sutra. You will learn techniques that have aroused the sex lives of couples over the centuries and gain a more thorough understanding of what Kama Sutra really teaches, apart from just the lovemaking secrets.

Don't delay your path to a more intimate, pleasurable and lasting sex life with your significant other. Start reading today and become the ultimate lover, ready to blow your partner's mind.

Chapter One: History And Philosophy Of Kama Sutra

For much of the Western world, the Kama Sutra is perceived to be mainly a sex guide. Although there are plenty of explicit sexual techniques presented in the Kama Sutra, only about 20% of the text actually discusses sexual techniques and positions. A bigger chunk of the text revolves around the path towards a life of virtue and grace as it relates to love, family, sex, relationships, and the human experience in general. Most of the Kama Sutra compares and contrasts various human desires, as well as the positive and negative effects of desire.

Scholars and historians maintain that the Kama Sutra was first written between 400 BC and 200 AD. The Kama Sutra in its current form was collated around 200 AD. The Indian philosopher Vatsyayana was the author of the Kama Sutra, and the writings themselves are part of a wider group of ancient Sanskrit writings called the Kama Shastra. Vatsyayana credits other Sanskrit writers' works as basis for his own Kama Sutra compilation, including those of Dattaka, Suvarnanabha, Ghotakamukha, Charayana and others.

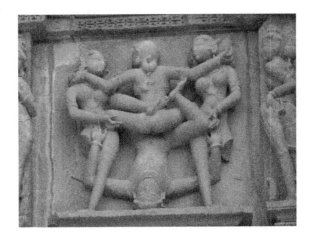

The Kama Sutra text contains 1250 verses, divided into 36 chapters, and structured into seven general sections, namely: **General Remarks**, containing the goals and priorities of life, gaining knowledge and proper conduct; **Sexual Stimulation and Union**, with techniques on sexual stimulation, caressing, kissing, positions, oral sex and other sexual techniques; **Getting a Wife**, with instructions on courting a girl, different types of marriage, etc.; **The Responsibilities of the Wife**; **The Behavior of Other Wives or Concubines**; **Advice for Courtesans**; and **Using Occult Techniques for Better Sexual Attraction**.

In the Kama Sutra, Vatsyayana sought to highlight, or extol, the attainment of a virtuous life and how human desires are interconnected to this aim. The word Kama in Sanskrit means desire, and while this could pertain to sexual desire, the word may also refer to love, affection, wishes, or aesthetic or physical stimulation, not necessarily sexual in nature. Kama is one of the four main goals of life in ancient Indian philosophy, the rest of which are dharma (or virtue), artha (money and possessions), and moksha (freedom from the cycle of reincarnation).

The Kama Sutra teaches concepts on the pleasures of sensual living in general, based heavily on other Indian writings as compiled by Vatsyayana, himself a philosopher from northern India. For Vatsyayana, the study of sexual knowledge was a form of meditation, spirituality and oneness with deity. Although the text deals with many other topics, it is the sexual techniques of the Kama Sutra that have garnered the most mainstream attention.

According to the Kama Sutra, a marriage will be happier and more fulfilling if both the husband and the wife have gained a lot of knowledge and skills in the areas of physical and mental pleasures. The text consistently teaches that in the art of lovemaking, the mind and the body are intertwined, and for total intimacy and sexual compatibility to be achieved, both the mind and the body should be working closely together.

Much of the sexually explicit methods that have embodied most people's notions on the Kama Sutra are found in the second section, or the ten chapters dealing with sexual stimulation, desire, copulation, and acts. These chapters depict a wide range of sexual acts incorporating different techniques of kissing, biting, embracing, scratching, oral sex, intercourse, and foreplay.

The Kama Sutra is a notable work of literature in that it is unabashedly contrary to much of the Western mores and ideals regarding marriage and sexuality. While monogamy in committed relationships is extolled today, the Kama Sutra embodies the more liberated societal realities of ancient Indian Hindu philosophy. The Kama Sutra has an entire category dealing with the courtesan and how she can gratify her man, and chapters that discuss the relationship of the husband, the wife, and the concubines or other wives, a concept which is taboo in most Western cultures today.

Philosophies in the Kama Sutra often appear to be strikingly discordant, and yet somehow cohesive in their entirety. The Kama Sutra, for instance, has two chapters that deal mainly with the responsibilities and the benefits of the wife, while also discussing how the 'main wife' will deal with the concubines. The chapters on concubines and courtesans all somehow are covered extensively, but without diminishing the importance of the woman's pleasure. In particular, the Kama Sutra teaches that it is the man's responsibility to satisfy his wife's sexual desires, and if she does not gain this satisfaction from him, she may seek pleasure from someone else.

There have been numerous translations and compilations of the Kama Sutra texts through the ages. One of the most notable was the Ananga-Ranga, which was composed in the 15th century and is a revised version of Vatsyayana's original writings. However, because it was written in Sanskrit which is quite difficult to comprehend, translate faithfully, and study, the Kama Sutra became obscure for many centuries.

The Kama Sutra resurfaced in mainstream consciousness sometime in the late 19th century when Arabic translator and linguist Sir Richard

Burton started on a translation of the Ananga-Ranga. Sir Burton's research into the Ananga-Ranga led him to unearth the original writings of Vatsyayana's Kama Sutra. Eventually, Sir Burton's work with Indian archaeologist Bhagwan Lal Indraji, Indian government officer Forster Fitzgerald Arbuthnot, and student Shivaram Parshuram Bhide led to the printing of an English translation of the Kama Sutra in 1883.

There have been various translations and revisions of the Kama Sutra in English; but to this day, Sir Burton's published version is still regarded as among the most accurate and faithful to the original text. Other noteworthy translations of the Kama Sutra include the work of Indra Sinha (1980), which contains the chapter on sexual acts many today associate with the text, and 1994's The Complete Kama Sutra by Alain Danielou. Danielou's work is noted for its use of original references to sex organs, and the use of original Sanskrit words in more contemporary contexts.

Is the Kama Sutra a guidebook for tantric sex? Tantric sex has a mixture of New Age and modern Western concepts interspersed with Buddhist and Hindu tantra and is nowadays synonymous with sexual practices and techniques that promote an elevated level of spirituality and sensual awareness. While there are some similarities and common concepts with tantric yoga, Kama Sutra is not a manual for tantric sex, contrary to many peoples' perception.

It is important to understand that the text of the Kama Sutra related to sexual activities are ultimately tied to its philosophy that human desires can be used to unleash a person's full potential, all with the goal of achieving virtuous living. The Kama Sutra does not contain practices or rituals that are tantric in nature, and it does not consider itself to be a sacred text for sexual rituals. In its philosophy, Kama Sutra is more humanistic, which sets it apart from the spirituality of tantric sexual practices.

Why has the Kama Sutra enamoured couples, lovers, and enthusiasts for generations? What are the advantages that this collection of ancient Sanskrit text can add to your sexual prowess or passion? In the next chapter, let us consider some of the appealing benefits that the Kama Sutra can offer to you and your partner as you ignite your bedroom activity and rekindle those passionate encounters.

Chapter Summary

- The Kama Sutra, although known primarily as a sex guide, revolves around the ancient Hindu philosophies of achieving life's goals through virtue.
- The original texts of the Kama Sutra were written between 400 BC to 200 AD. Much of the text we know today was compiled by Vatsyayana, an Indian philosopher and monk.
- The Kama Sutra is divided into seven sections and has 1250 verses grouped into 36 chapters.
- Only 20% of the Kama Sutra, just one section, discusses explicit sexual techniques. Other sections discuss proper conduct, reaching life's goals and priorities, types of marriage, rules for the wife, and instructions for concubines and courtesans, among other topics.
- The main tenet of the sexual lessons found in the Kama Sutra is the importance of knowledge and skills in the area of lovemaking, as a component to a happy marriage or partnership.
- In the Kama Sutra, it is the man or the husband's duty to provide sexual pleasure to his wife.
- Various English translations of the Kama Sutra have been published since the 19th century.
- Kama Sutra is different from tantric sex and should not be misconstrued as a manual for such.

Chapter Two: Benefits Of The Kama Sutra

It is interesting how the Kama Sutra has survived thousands of years and continues to be relevant and useful to modern-day readers. Even with the advent of technology and the many innovations and discoveries regarding human sexuality and interactions, there is something about the ancient texts of the Kama Sutra that still rings true to its followers today.

In many ways, the Kama Sutra was ahead of its time and is still quite bold and out-of-the-box in its views regarding sexuality and pleasure. Whereas much of the major religions and societal structures and mores have restricted open discussions on sexuality, relegating it to hushed dialogues or backroom whispers, the Kama Sutra fully embraced sexual pleasure as part of a healthy life. It promoted the idea that a person who is comfortable with himself or herself sexually, will also have a more balanced, well-rounded, and happy life.

The Kama Sutra also placed sexuality on a pedestal by teaching that sexual pleasure is a vital ingredient to married life. In stark contrast, many cultures and eras have often viewed sex as a necessary evil or only as a means for procreation and the continued propagation of the human race. Little regard was given to whether the man or woman's sexual appetites were being satisfied. In the Kama Sutra, however, sexual gratification for both partners is celebrated, studied, and fully explored in all its naked glory.

As is the case with any work of literature or prevailing school of thought, myths and misconceptions around the Kama Sutra have often blurred its essence, especially as it experienced a resurgence and caught a wider audience in the Western world. Many view the Kama Sutra as just a guide for different sex positions and techniques, or as a manual for teaching the man or the woman different styles of foreplay, intercourse, and everything else in between. While the Kama Sutra does teach all of these, it goes beyond just the physical aspect of lovemaking. In fact, it treats lovemaking as an art, just like music, sculpture, or painting, with layers of intricacies and painstaking detail given to producing a masterpiece.

One of the biggest benefits of the Kama Sutra is its focus on bringing couples and partners closer to each other. Intimacy plays an important role in the celebration of sexuality in the context of the Kama Sutra, as it endeavors to make readers comfortable in their own skin. The Kama Sutra is an excellent way for couples to open up to each other and begin to communicate more seamlessly about their sexual urges, needs and sweet spots, all with the goal of satisfying one another.

Inevitably, as the Kama Sutra journey commences, partners become closer to each other as they also grow more aware of what the other person is thinking, feeling, and wanting. Sex, after all, can be a uniquely intimate expression of love and affection between two committed individuals, and the techniques depicted in the Kama Sutra help to further enhance the close relationship of two people wanting to satisfy each other in the bedroom. Learning the Kama Sutra techniques together means making discoveries, committing mistakes, and achieving new heights of ecstasy with your significant other, and this can solidify the bond that has already formed.

Another benefit of the Kama Sutra is its detailed teachings on oral sex. Fellatio and cunnilingus tips are dished out in the Kama Sutra and considered an intrinsic part of the art of lovemaking. While it is true that many people today are aware of oral sex and can perform it on their partner, many are unaware that there are strategies that can make the experience even more pleasurable, thus exciting and satisfying the other person beyond just the ordinary.

Also, considered a fringe benefit of learning the techniques given in the Kama Sutra, comes a boost of confidence and self-esteem for both partners in the relationship. When you realize that you are giving your spouse or partner wild orgasms or reaching the throes of sexual climax unlike ever before, this can elevate your confidence to higher levels as

93

well. The Kama Sutra provides techniques on lasting longer and being able to make each lovemaking session more extended and packed with more action, so you can hone your skills and become that unforgettable lover you have always aspired to be.

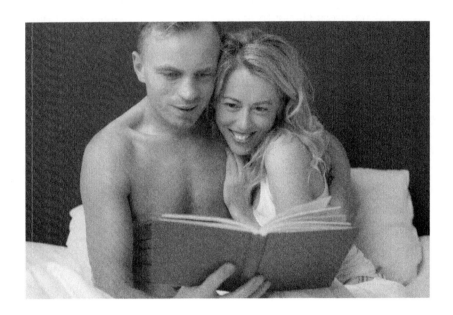

In relationships, the partner who is more attuned to the physical, emotional, and sexual needs of the other person increases his or her attractiveness. This is because you are able to reach those urges and cravings of the other person, and the fulfilment of these wants and needs becomes congruent to your attentiveness and ability to perform. Think about how memorable and sexually attractive you will become to your spouse or partner if you are the only one able to give them that intense sexual climax or mind-blowing foreplay they thought only existed in their wildest imagination? The Kama Sutra tenets increase your mutual attraction and will heat things up in the bedroom.

The Kama Sutra has a very positive, empowering, and healthy view of human sexuality, and it can help you or your partner overcome any negative perceptions, hang-ups, or experiences with sex. Many people are unable to fully enjoy their sexual appetite because of previous bad notions, misconceptions, or wrong expectations, and the Kama Sutra writings can help in correcting these misconstrued views and cultivate a healthier attitude towards this act.

As already mentioned, the Kama Sutra is far from just a sex guide that espouses emotionless intercourse between two individuals. Rather, it recognizes that the pleasures of sexual intimacy start in the minds and spirits of participants, so there are discussions in the ancient writings that deal with developing a closer relationship to each other. When the emotional connection is nurtured, conversations become more open and honest, and sexual compatibility also heightens. At the same time, when sexual gratification is fulfilled for both partners, the emotional and mental bonds are also fully engaged, improving the state of the relationship as a whole.

For the purposes of this book, however, we will focus mainly on the sexual aspects embodied in the writings of the Kama Sutra. In the next chapter, you will read about the foreplay techniques in the Kama Sutra, and its importance in the art of lovemaking. How do you heat things up in the bedroom through thorough, thoughtful and titillating foreplay skills? Read on to find out.

Chapter Summary

- Despite being written centuries ago the Kama Sutra is still as relevant to today's society.
- The writings of the Kama Sutra celebrate and embrace human sexuality as a healthy and normal part of life.
- More than just the sexual techniques, the Kama Sutra presents lovemaking as an art, not any different from music, painting, or sculpture.
- The Kama Sutra can help bring couples closer to each other, foster deeper conversations, and strengthen emotional connections.
- Successful application of the Kama Sutra techniques can elevate one's self-confidence as a lover and increase attractiveness.
- Oral sex techniques are discussed in detail in the Kama Sutra with the goal of pleasuring one's partner beyond their imagination.
- The ancient Kama Sutra texts promote a healthy and empowering view of human sexuality, thus helping to transform negative perceptions of sex.

Chapter Three: Foreplay Techniques In The Kama Sutra

Foreplay is the appetizer to the main course. Many couples rush through foreplay or even skip it altogether, getting to the main dish right away. However, extended and intense foreplay sessions tend to heighten sexual pleasure for both partners and can make the experience even more memorable for both. In the Kama Sutra, particular attention is given to foreplay techniques because it can set the stage for a more explosive climax.

Why is foreplay important? You can think of the human body like a car engine. When your car has been parked overnight, the engine has cooled down substantially and needs a couple of minutes to warm up in order to run better. During colder months, you may need up to ten minutes to warm up your car before hitting the road. You will notice the difference in performance between a car that has been properly warmed up against a car that is started and driven without ample time for the engine to get things warmed up inside.

In the same way, the human body performs better when it has been revved up substantially, and foreplay does this job. Men need to understand this part of the lovemaking process particularly because their female partner needs foreplay to really enjoy sex. Dr. Ruth Westheimer, a psychosexual therapist and professor/lecturer at New York University, Yale, and Princeton, notes, "It's particularly important for women to have successful foreplay because it takes a woman a longer time than a man to get up to the level of arousal needed to orgasm."

Men take a shorter time to become sexually aroused. In fact, a lot of men walk around with sex on their minds constantly and may only need a couple of minutes to be ready for action. Women, however, are wired differently and may need more attentive and thoughtful foreplay to be ready for sex. The female body needs not just the physical aspect, but also the emotional and mental preparation, and intense foreplay can open this portal in the female sexual experience more than any other aspect of lovemaking. Copious amounts of kissing, hugging, touching, caressing, and other foreplay induces the vagina to create lubrication, making sexual intercourse more comfortable and pleasurable.

Foreplay fulfills a dual purpose. It encourages blood flow to the penis, making it erect and ready for intercourse and makes the blood flow to the clitoris in much the same way as the penis. When blood flows to the clitoris, it becomes erect and more sensitive. An erect clitoris can be stimulated to achieve pleasure. Foreplay lubricates the vagina and hardens the clitoris, and this combination can make the sexual encounter more pleasurable for the woman.

Foreplay also gives the woman the emotional assurance she needs. The woman needs to be reminded that the man is not just having sex with her to satisfy his own needs, but because he genuinely cares for her and wants to spend time with her while being attentive to her sexual needs. When foreplay is extended, skillful and imaginative, it gives the woman the confidence that she has the full attention of her partner.

Kissing

For most couples, foreplay starts with kissing. Kissing can be done in certain types of techniques and positions on the lips and the body to create sexual tension. Specific zones of the body can turn on your partner quite significantly if you kiss the right area. Sensitive areas your partner will get turned on by are the Lips, Neck, Stomach and Inner thigh. Here are some of the main types of kissing as described in the Kama Sutra:

The Measured Kiss. This kiss refers to one partner offering their lips to be kissed but without moving them. The other partner will actively kiss the mouth while one remains passive.

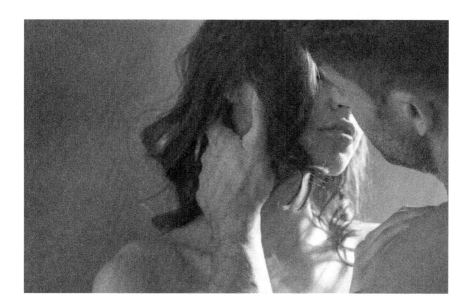

The Throbbing Kiss. In the throbbing kiss, the lips of both partners will touch, but only their lower lips will move. This may happen at the start of foreplay when the woman is still a bit shy and needs some prodding to release passion.

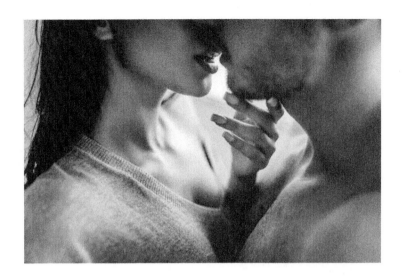

The Direct Kiss. As things heat up, excitement builds, and the direct kiss can be added. In this kiss, both partners face each other, press their mouths together, and begin to lick and suck each other's lips and mouths. Some biting may be incorporated.

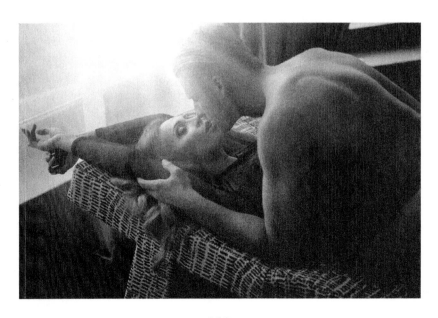

The Pressure Kiss. Couples who enjoy some aggressive foreplay can try the pressure kiss, where one partner keeps the other partner's mouth and lips closed while biting, kissing, and licking passionately. Holding their arms down against the bed or a wall will induce more sexual tension also

The Contact Kiss. In this kiss, one partner teases the other with a light, provocative kiss that only lightly touches the mouth. The partner then holds back while staring into the others eyes creating sexual tension from the get go.

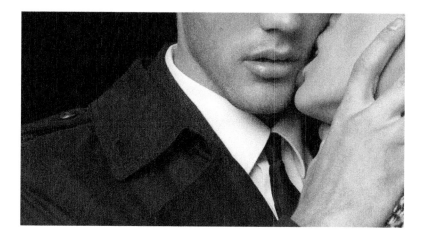

The Kiss To Ignite Flame. This kiss seems innocent but is designed to awaken the other partner's sexual mood. It is often used to determine if the other partner is still up for sexual activity. In this kiss, one partner innocently but seductively plants a kiss on the other partner's (passive) lips, usually while the partner is sleeping or resting, and waits for a response to determine if sexual activity will be welcomed.

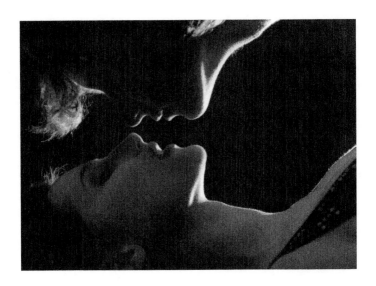

The Distraction Kiss. This kiss is not limited to the mouth. Rather, it can be used to warm up your partner by also directing attention to other parts of the body, such as the face, ears, chest, nape, neck, or shoulders. Many of these areas have very sensitive nerve endings and are called erogenous zones.

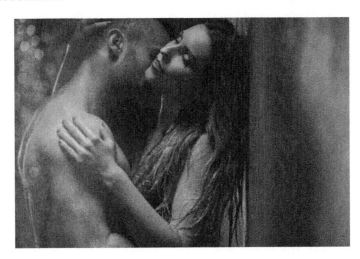

The Finger Kiss. A precursor to oral sex, this kiss involves putting one's finger in the other partner's mouth, with some movements inside, and then removing the finger and brushing it across the lips.

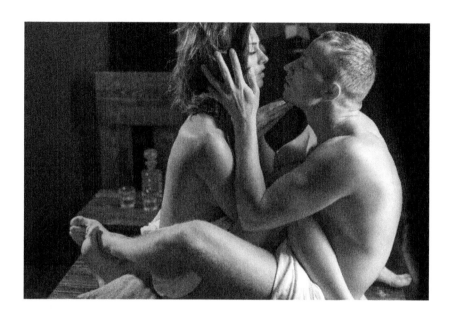

Touching And Body Massage

Aside from the intense and varied embraces and kisses in the Kama Sutra, attention is also given to other forms of body touching and massaging. Massaging can be especially relaxing and arousing to both the male and the female, and can be a loving, soothing precursor to the lovemaking session. In the Kama Sutra, these types of body massage are taught:

Face Down. This usually starts with a shoulder press, with the partner lying down on their stomach, while the other partner sits on their back and starts massaging the shoulders, loosening up the body and moving down.

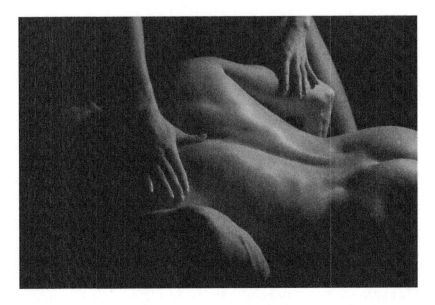

Rake Touch. As the body's muscles slowly relax and release tension, the fingers may now be moved lightly up and down the torso. This can be extremely sensual and sometimes quite ticklish for others. For added excitement, you may also use your lips or tongue to follow the same path that your fingers travel

Back Massage. The back massage must be done firmly but without digging into the body with the fingernails. The palms must slide and knead the skin and muscles both gently and firmly, with just the right amount of pressure. Strokes are done slowly and rhythmically, especially in the lower back and shoulders. For males, the lower back is an erogenous zone, while for females, the shoulders are particularly excitable. During the back massage, special attention should be given to the region between the buttocks and the spine known as the sacrum. This area is very sensitive to touch, and massaging this area with small, circular, rhythmic strokes down to the buttocks and thighs can heighten sexual arousal.

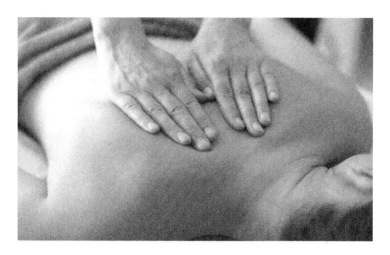

Thigh Massage. Keeping the hands well-lubricated, massage the upper and lower thighs with gentle kneading and stroking. This area is also very sensitive to touch, especially within the insides of the leg.

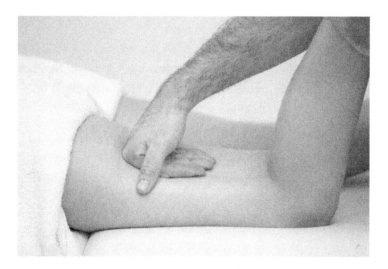

Release Points Massage. The neck, ears, and chest or breasts are erogenous zones for males and females. Small circular massages around these release points can arouse the partner.

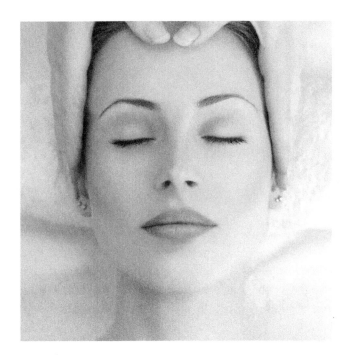

As you follow these Kama Sutra techniques on kissing, embracing, and touching, the sexual excitement will continue to increase. In the next chapter, you will read about the holy grail of female sexual organs – the clitoris. The Kama Sutra knows the intense power of this small but significant part of the female anatomy, and we will uncover its secrets.

Chapter Summary

- Think of lovemaking as a full-course meal, with foreplay as the appetizer.
- Long, thoughtful, pleasurable foreplay sessions add to the excitement of the lovemaking and build up the body to a more powerful climax.
- For females, foreplay is especially important because it induces vaginal lubrication and makes intercourse more pleasurable.
- In males, exquisite foreplay enhances the erection, while in females, it encourages the flow of blood to the clitoris.
- The Kama Sutra discusses several forms of kissing and embracing, all with varying degrees of passion and intensity, that are part of the foreplay.
- Foreplay is not limited to the bedroom. Throughout the day, couples may engage in foreplay and build up towards the grand finale in the evening.
- Body massage is also an integral part of Kama Sutra-style sex, with special attention given to sexual release points in the body.

Chapter Four: Clitoral Stimulation For Female Orgasms

As society has become more open to sexuality, women have also been encouraged to talk more about their sexual desires and needs. Men have always been quite vocal about their sexual gratification, but for most cultures women are not as frank in discussing what they like in bed. The sexual revolution of recent decades has opened the floodgates for more engaging conversations on the female body as it relates to sexual activity.

The clitoris as a female sexual organ has received a lot of mainstream attention, and yet continues to be shrouded in a lot of mystery. This female body part is still largely misunderstood by the male gender and often overlooked. Women, however, have become more aware of the promise of pleasure that can be delivered by the clitoris.

Situated at the top region of the female vulva, or external female genitalia, the clitoris has two main parts, namely the glans and the shaft. The glans is external and visible, about the size of a pearl, while the shaft is an internal part of the clitoris about one inch in length and running upwards from the glans. The clitoris has a piece of skin known as the clitoral hood which fully or partially hides it. Female natural secretions keep the hood lubricated over the clitoris.

The clitoris contains more nerve endings than any other part of the female anatomy. It is highly sensitive to touch or stimulation. When the female becomes sexually aroused, blood begins to flow to the clitoris, and it expands in size and becomes more erect, similar to the male penis (but substantially smaller). Clitoral stimulation is the surest way for the female to achieve orgasm or sexual climax, compared to vaginal penetration. In fact, the clitoris has no other function in the body other than sexual arousal. It is there precisely to enhance pleasure in the female, which is why it should be studied closely by any lover who wishes to cause toe-curling orgasms in their female partner.

You should note that the clitoris, being very sensitive, is a part of the body which some women would rather have indirectly stimulated than directly. The lips, tongue, fingers, hands, and penis may be used for clitoral stimulation. In the Kama Sutra, some techniques involve manual stimulation of the clitoris with the use of the fingers. You may start with one finger, then two fingers, with circular rubbing movements around the clitoris as the female adjusts to the sensation. Pressure and speed may be increased as the woman becomes more aroused.

During cunnilingus, or oral sex, the clitoris may also be directly or indirectly stimulated. The partner may lick or suck on the clitoris, stimulating the thousands of nerve endings in this body part, until the clitoris becomes fully erect. The clitoris may also be directly or indirectly stimulated during intercourse, as certain positions, such as the missionary, rubs against the pubic bone and indirectly, the clitoris. Whatever sexual position is being performed, either one of the partners may rub the clitoris during intercourse to heighten female pleasure.

Clitoris Stimulating Sex Positions

In the Kama Sutra, the following sexual positions are depicted as the most pleasurable for women specifically because of the clitoral stimulation involved:

The Mold. This position pertains to the man lying astride the woman and entering her from the side, which allows him to fondle her breasts, kiss her lips and face, and to rub the clitoris during penetration. This position is especially suitable for couples where the man is heavier, and the woman cannot support his weight. The angle also allows for deeper and more thorough penetration, intensifying the sensation for the man, while at the same time allowing him or the woman to access the clitoris or the breasts for female climax.

For women who like to have their neck, nape, ears, shoulders, or upper back kissed or licked during sex, the Mold position is particularly enticing. These erogenous zones are available to the man's mouth and tongue in this angle, and the man can send her to an explosive climax by stimulating her clitoris and nipples and kissing her neck while thrusting into her, all at the same time. The woman, on the other hand, can move her hands around his arms, head, or grip his buttocks during penetration, guiding the speed and depth.

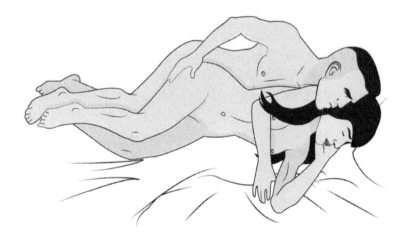

Face To Face. In this position, both partners are facing each other, with the female positioned on top of the man, and penetration is gentler but directly stimulates much of the front areas of the vagina, including the clitoris. As the thrusting increases in speed, so does the stimulation to the clitoris. Additionally, the man is free to caress or stimulate other areas of the woman's body. He can grip her buttocks, stroke her back, while she controls the speed and depth of the penetration.

Couples where the woman has a smaller vagina in relation to his penis would find this position suitable because she can control the depth of the penetration especially at the beginning of the intercourse. For women with smaller vaginas, the initial penetration needs to be done gently and slowly at first, allowing her organ to slowly expand and receive the penis. Because she is in control, she can relax her muscles and slowly guide him inside her, controlling the tempo until he is fully inside. As the intercourse ensues, the natural lubrication secreted from the vagina will make penetration more pleasurable for both partners.

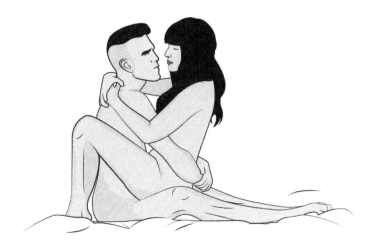

Missionary. This sexual position is arguably the most popular of all, and the easiest for both partners. At the same time, it involves a lot of friction in the pelvic regions and can be very pleasurable for females. In the classic missionary position, the woman lies on her back as the man gets on top of her, between her thighs, and commences penetration. During intercourse, the woman can focus on her pleasure, and the clitoris is also accessible to both partners for manual stimulation. Women particularly enjoy this position because aside from the clitoral stimulation from the pelvis, there is face-to-face contact and a closer emotional connection to the man. Keep in mind that for females, sex is just as much an emotional as well as physical activity, and the sight of their partner on top of them, intertwined with their body, is a major turn-on for women.

Another advantage of the missionary position is it allows the couple to better angle the penetration, usually by adding a pillow underneath the woman's buttocks, to increase the stimulation of the clitoris during intercourse. This can be achieved without necessarily adding strain to either the man's or the woman's movements. Of course, as this happens, the friction intensifies, increasing the pleasure for the woman, while the man can thrust deeper into her nether regions, increasing the penile sensations as well.

The missionary position is one of the most intimate sexual positions in the Kama Sutra, and it remains to be among the most popular among couples, especially those in committed and long-term relationships. The missionary position allows for a lot of eye contact and is both physically pleasurable and highly affectionate. Kissing, caressing, light biting or spanking, and other sexual actuations may also be added to this position to increase sensations. Couples who enjoy a little bit of consensual domination or role-play may add blindfolding, tying, handcuffs, or ankle straps to the missionary position for variety.

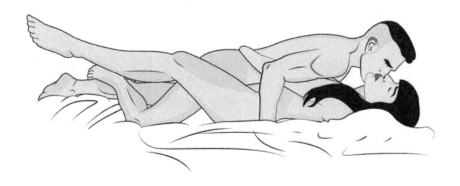

Delight. This position is often depicted in mainstream media and is among the most pleasurable for both males and females. The position refers to the woman sitting up and the man kneeling in between her thighs, embracing her around the back, while her legs straddle him. The angle of the penetration ensures constant clitoral stimulation, and the man is also free to stroke her breasts or kiss her upper body while penetrating the vagina. The Delight position is very erotic and sensual for couples. This position is particularly suitable for couples where the woman is too small to carry the weight of the man.

The delight position is also very intimate, like the missionary position, because it allows for a lot of eye-to-eye contact. As the bodies are more closely intertwined to each other, the emotional connection is also greater during intercourse. The woman can communicate to the man what other areas of her body she would like to be stimulated during this position, and he is free to kiss her ears, neck, nape, shoulders, and other areas of her upper body, while his hands can move around her back, buttocks, waist, hips, and other parts.

As mentioned in the earlier part of this chapter, the clitoris may be directly stimulated using the tongue, lips, or mouth aside from the hands or fingers. In the next chapter, we will discuss more of this in detail as we delve into the oral sex techniques put forth in the ancient texts of the Kama Sutra.

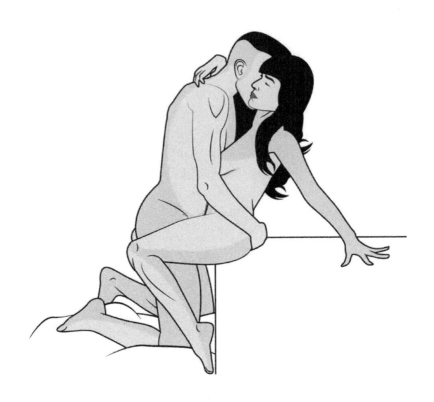

Chapter Summary

- The clitoris is found in the top area of the vulva, and consists of the glans (visible), the shaft (internal), and the clitoral hood (skin covering).
- The clitoris contains thousands of nerve endings and is the most sensitive part of the female body.
- Clitoral stimulation is the surest way to achieve female orgasm, more than vaginal penetration.
- The clitoris may be stimulated manually, during intercourse, or during cunnilingus.

Chapter Five: Oral Sex Techniques In The Kama Sutra

Oral sex may be part of the foreplay but may also be performed at any time during the lovemaking session of a couple. In fact, some couples may find it enjoyable to alternate between bouts of foreplay, penetration, oral sex, and other acts. There is no set rule that says oral sex should only be done before intercourse or as part of foreplay.

In the Kama Sutra, philosopher Vatsyayana discussed oral sex techniques in detail as part of continued experimentation and exploration of partners and couples. At the same time, Vatsyayana also wrote the text in the context of society at the time, where harems of the rulers had many kept women and oral sex was one of the methods used to avoid pregnancy.

Female Oral Techniques & Positions

Fellatio

Let us first look at some Kama Sutra techniques for fellatio, or oral sex performed on the male. Known in colloquial usage as a blowjob, fellatio is highly pleasurable for the man and can intensify sexual excitement.

Touching. This fellatio technique is described as the woman holding the penis in her hand, forming a letter 'O' with her lips, then touching them to the tip of the penis. Then, she moves her head in tiny circular motions. In this movement, her lips and tongue will focus pleasure on the glans or 'head' of the penis which is extremely sensitive, thus increasing his libido and preparing his erection for penetration. This technique is also called Nimitta and is a great first step for beginners who are giving fellatio for the first time.

During fellatio, the woman should be careful not to accidentally graze her teeth against the head or the sides of the penis as this can be painful. While some men do enjoy the sensation of light biting along the penis shaft, teeth grazing the penis especially during up and down movements can be painful. This is the reason for the 'O' shape which she forms with her lips, thus keeping the teeth behind the lips and away from his member.

Nominal Congress. In this oral sex technique, the woman holds the penis with one hand, places the penis between her lips, and then moves her mouth in a mild, gentle motion around the head of the penis. The nerve endings of the tip of the penis are very sensitive and this technique can be very sensual and ticklish. Again, the woman should be careful not to let her teeth graze the head of the penis. One technique that can be added to this fellatio style is licking the slit or the inside of the penis head. This area is very sensitive and can drive the man to near-orgasmic pleasure.

When performing this fellatio technique, the woman can think of how she eats a lollipop or ice popsicle. The movement is mild, a bit circular, and with the lips applying most of the pressure while the tongue is used to taste the penis as it is inside the mouth. Pay close attention to the tip of the glans and the sides of the head. The other hand not holding the penis may be used to stimulate the man's nipples or scrotum.

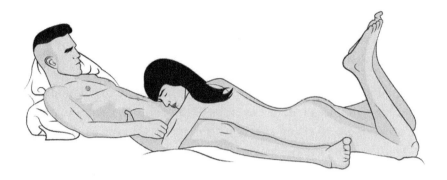

Parshvatoddashta. This technique is translated as biting the sides, where the partner grasps the head of the penis firmly, clamping her lips around the shaft, then moving from one side to the other, taking care not to bite into the penis with her teeth. The shaft will be gently caressed by her lips and tongue, creating an intense sensation for the male. The lips of the woman are particularly pleasurable to the man's penis because this closely resembles the vagina. In fact, many men find the mouth to be more pleasurable because it is more lubricated (due to the saliva), and because of the suction which can be performed by the partner giving fellatio. In this technique, the penis also probes the sides of the mouth, inside the cheeks, and the sensation can drive the man wild.

For women who have a gag reflex and find it difficult to take in more of the penis in their mouth, or if the man has a particularly large penis which is difficult to take in fully, this technique is suitable to try because it targets the sides rather than the inner mouth or throat of the woman.

Bahiha-samdansha. This fellatio technique pertains to taking the head of the penis between the lips, pressing it tenderly, and pulling at the soft skin under the head of the penis. This skin is very sensitive, so the woman should take care not to bite hard, only applying enough pressure to be able to pull the skin and play with it using her mouth. For men who are uncircumcised, many of the nerve endings connecting this area to the foreskin are extremely sensitive and can intensify sexual arousal by leaps and bounds.

This fellatio technique has the additional sensation of teasing the penis of the man in an area that is integral to sexual climax, but without necessarily moving the mouth in a way that will bring him closer to ejaculation. The teasing sensation can drive him wild and make the woman feel more dominant because she holds his sexual release in her hands, literally.

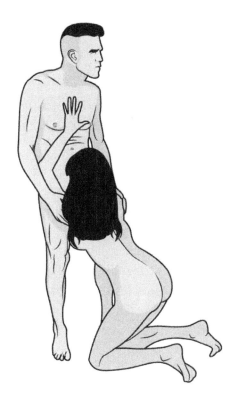

Antaha-samdansha. Similar to the technique above, this is also called the inner pincer. The woman lets the head of the penis slide fully into her mouth, then she presses the shaft of the penis with her lips, staying there for a few minutes before pulling away. The depth, pressure, and speed will increase as arousal intensifies. The man will feel his sexual excitement increasing as he gets close to the edge, only to be denied release as the woman presses the shaft of the penis, thus delaying his climax. As the climax is delayed, the penis becomes more erect and ready for vaginal penetration. The more rigid the penis when penetration ensues, the more pleasurable the sensations will be for the woman.

Chumbitaka. This pertains to kissing the penis as you would the mouth. The partner takes the penis in her hand, rounds her lips, then kisses the length of the penis while gently stroking. This technique explores the length of the penis, not just the head. As the woman's lips travel down the length of the shaft, she can use her lips to perform small sucking movements on the sides of the penis, while stroking the head or using her other hand to also lightly massage the scrotum. Many women are not aware that while much of the sensations are centered on the head of the penis, the shaft is also sensitive and needs attention during fellatio.

Parimrshtaka. This technique makes use of the woman's tongue, repeatedly flicking and striking the tip of the glans of the penis. Keep in mind that this is a very sensitive area, and some men may take a while to get used to the sensation. Other may find it too painful. The man must clearly communicate to the woman what is pleasurable for him in this technique and what he finds too painful. For most men, however, the tip of the glans can be stimulated with the tongue so long as it is done very gently and slowly at first, increasing in intensity as he gets used to the sensation. The slit is very sensitive especially when flicked with the tongue over and over.

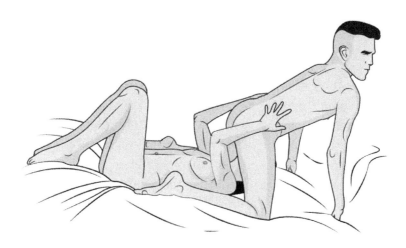

Sucking A Mango Fruit. Referred to in the Kama Sutra as Amrachushita, this technique refers to taking the penis deeply into the mouth, pulling and sucking vigorously as if sucking the mango seed. The sucking motion coupled with the sensation of the erect penis being fully enveloped by the mouth of the woman is extremely pleasurable to the man and can increase arousal, perhaps even bring the man close to a climax.

The woman can also use her free hands to stimulate other areas of the man's body, such as the nipples. The feeling of having the nipples stimulated lightly while receiving fellatio is very intense for the man. The woman can also roam her hands along the length of his body or use her fingers to play with his scrotum or the area between the scrotum and the anus. Many men also enjoy having their anus stimulated during fellatio, especially while the penis is being sucked deeply.

Sangara. This pertains to allowing the man to ejaculate into the mouth of the woman, using the lips and tongue to suck the penis until orgasm is achieved. The sensation will be very intense, and for many men the feeling of their intimate bodily fluid being taken in the mouth by their partner is an intimate and deeply personal act.

Some women, however, may not be comfortable taking the man's ejaculate into their mouth, so this should be discussed prior to oral sex. The man's semen contains the sperm cells, but also about 200 different types of proteins, vitamins, and minerals, including vitamin C, calcium, citric acid, fructose, lactic acid, magnesium, phosphorus, potassium, sodium, vitamin B12, and zinc. A teaspoon of semen, which is the normal amount excreted during ejaculation, contains between 5-25 calories, and the level of the compounds differs based on diet, exercise, age, weight, and other lifestyle choices. The fluid, then, is safe for the female partner to take in her mouth if she is comfortable doing so.

Male Oral Techniques & Positions

Cunnilingus

Known in modern terms as "giving head", cunnilingus is an act that the male partner must master because it can deliver massive waves of orgasm to the female. Here are some cunnilingus techniques taught in the Kama Sutra:

Quivering Kiss. In this technique, the partner pinches the vagina's labia, shaping them like the lips, and then gently kissing the area as you would the mouth. This is called the Adhara-sphuritam in the Kama Sutra. The technique is very sensual and intimate, and some women with more sensitive labia may find the pinching a bit uncomfortable at first. If this is the case, initial pinching should be done gently at first, allowing the woman to become more comfortable with the sensation.

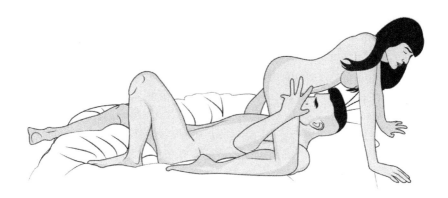

Circling Tongue. The Kama Sutra calls this Jihva-bhramanaka and refers to spreading the lips of the vagina and using the tongue to probe inside as the nose, lips, and chin perform a slow circular movement. The vagina is very sensitive, so this technique should be done gently. The man is advised to shave prior to cunnilingus to lessen the irritation that the female may experience when the vagina comes into direct contact with facial hair.

As the sensation becomes more intense and the man's tongue probes faster, the woman may want to hold the back of her partner's head and guide him towards areas where she experiences more pleasure. During this technique, the man may also use his free hand to circle her nipples, or caress her ears, neck, lips, shoulders, legs, and other erogenous zones.

Tongue Massage. This cunnilingus technique involves touching the archway of the vagina with the tongue, then penetrating slowly, increasing the speed and rhythm, until the vagina produces lubrication. This is called Jihva-mardita in the ancient writings. The tongue massage is great for foreplay and relaxing the vagina for penetration and is also a very intimate activity that allows the man to inhale and taste the nether regions of his partner.

As the tongue massage is being given to her vagina, he may also use his hands to roam around her body, stimulating her nipples, hips, legs, buttocks, and other areas. The female may want to arch her back a little and allow the man's tongue to probe deeper into her pleasure zones. For maximum pleasure, the man may also use one hand to stimulate her clitoris as his tongue is probing her vagina. Not only does this bring the woman to a mind-blowing climax, but the combined lubrication of his saliva and her vaginal secretions make penetration easier and more pleasurable for both.

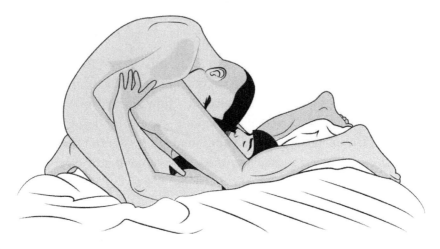

Sucking. Chushita, as it is called in the Kama Sutra, is the technique of fastening the lips to the vagina, then kissing deeply, nibbling, and sucking vigorously on the clitoris. As the man is kissing and sucking the clitoris and the outer areas of the vagina, he may also alternately probe the inner entryway of the vagina with his tongue or use his fingers to penetrate her vagina. This technique relaxes the vagina for penetration and is particularly useful for women with smaller vaginas. As the vagina relaxes and expands, it also secretes lubrication, it will be ready to receive the penis, thus making penetration more pleasurable for both partners.

Sucking Up. Uchchushita in the Kama Sutra, this means cupping the woman's buttocks and lifting up, then using the tongue to probe the navel down to the vagina, staying mostly in the external regions. Circular licking and sucking motions in the area between the navel and vagina are very stimulating to the female. Additionally, some women find the sensation of the man's facial hair stimulating their navel, penis, and outer vagina to be very pleasurable. Other women may find this too irritating, however, and it must be communicated clearly. Irritation can be lessened through proper shaving of facial hair.

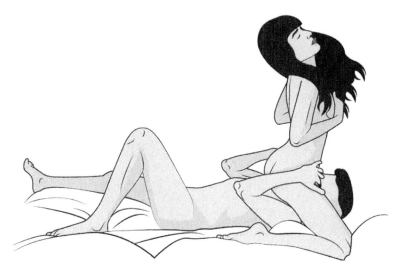

During uchchushita, the man may use his hands to travel around the woman's buttocks, occasionally moving up and down her back down to her thighs and legs. The woman, meanwhile, may use her hand to hold his nape and guide his mouth to areas where she feels the most sensations. The female can also move her pelvis in a rhythm to his sucking motions, focusing on her pleasure.

Stirring. In this style, the woman holds her thighs and spreads them apart as the partner uses his tongue to pleasure her inner thighs and vagina. The Kama Sutra calls this Kshobhaka. Adding the inner thighs to the stimulation of the vagina can be extremely pleasurable to the woman because the inner thighs are very sensitive erogenous zones. During stirring, the man may use his hands to travel the length of the woman's body or use his fingers to penetrate her vagina as he is pleasuring her inner thighs with his tongue.

For women who enjoy stimulation in or around the anus, this position opens up the anal area to the man's tongue, lips, and hands. The area just above the anus is especially pleasurable and becomes more accessible to the male partner as the woman holds her thighs.

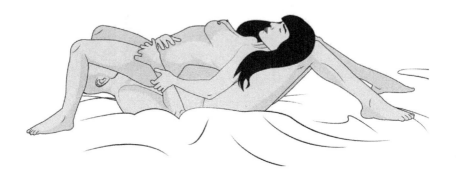

Sucking Hard. Called Bahuchushita in the ancient texts, this technique refers to setting the feet of the woman on the man's shoulders, clasping the hands around her waist, then sucking hard and long on her vaginal area as the tongue stirs inside. Couples who enjoy consensual domination or a little bit of role play will find this technique exciting, because the man now assumes the role of a slave who has no choice but to pleasure his female master with his oral skills. The weight of her feet on top of his shoulders may be moved closer to his neck, thus keeping his head in place and focusing on her pleasure.

In the bahuchushita position, the man's hands are on the woman's waist, where he is also free to move up and down the length of her torso. In this position, the woman's anus is also accessible to the man's tongue for stimulation, and if the woman particularly enjoys kissing in this area, she can let her partner know. The woman's hands, meanwhile, are free to stroke his hair, lift her leg up to make it easier for her partner or caress her own nipples and other erogenous zones as her feet keep his head around her nether regions.

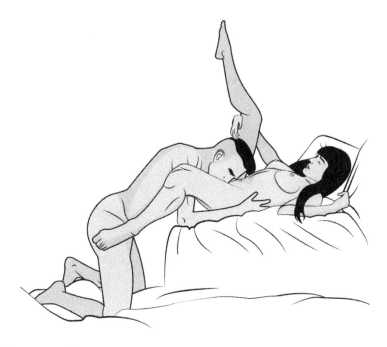

The Crow. In this cunnilingus technique, the couple lie side by side fronts toward each other, with one partners feet at the others' head, while kissing each other's private parts. This is also known as the Kakila and is quite similar to the 69-sexual position. The Kakila is highly erotic and allows the couple to stimulate each other orally at the same time. Both the man and the woman are giving and receiving oral sex, focusing on each other's sexual sensations, while also receiving pleasure for themselves.

The kakila position is particularly helpful for couples who want to try the 69-position but may be constrained by larger weight differences between the couple. For instance, the man may be too heavy for the woman to have to support with her weight. In the crow position, however, because both partners are side by side, supporting their weight is not an issue. Also, the playing field becomes more equal as no partner has the upper hand. With both partners next to each other, all erogenous zones are accessible for oral pleasure.

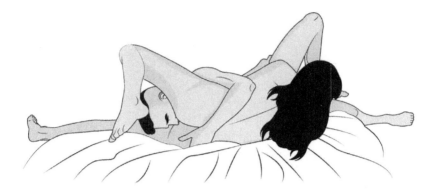

If weight or strength isn't a problem then the standard 69 position will be perfect because both partners get to enjoy the pleasure at the same time with their partners genitals deeply and perfectly inline for oral sex.

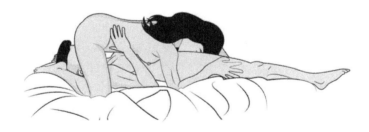

In oral sex, communication between the partners is very important. What is highly stimulating for one person may be uncomfortable for another individual. Some people have more sensitive endings in certain body parts than others, and this may require a gentler oral stimulation at first, building up to a crescendo of passion as the senses adjust.

As with any part of the Kama Sutra techniques, it is important that both partners are completely comfortable with themselves and each other, so letting your spouse or partner know what feels good and what does not is important. Instead of guessing or making your partner guess, be upfront and let them know what pushes your buttons. This is the goal of Kama Sutra, after all, which is to foster a more intimate relationship where both partners are attuned to each other's sexual desires and can give each other earth-shattering sexual climaxes because they already know what the other person needs.

After the oral sex practices given in the Kama Sutra, we now come to the sexual positions that the Kama Sutra is mostly known for today. In the next chapter, let us study some of the basic positions found in this ancient collection of texts.

Chapter Summary

- The Kama Sutra has many oral sex techniques designed for the mutual enjoyment and pleasure of sexual partners.
- Fellatio, or oral sex for the man, involves various styles that have varying degrees of pressure, speed, and motion.
- Cunnilingus, or oral sex for the woman, should be performed gently at first because the vagina is much more sensitive than the penis.
- Both partners are encouraged to clearly communicate what they like and do not like in oral sex. Some people's nether regions are more sensitive than others.
- Oral sex brings couples closer together and fosters a healthier, more intimately connected relationship.

Chapter Six: Beginner Sex Positions In The Kama Sutra

Aside from the Kama Sutra sex positions already discussed in the chapter on female clitoral stimulation, there are dozens of other sexual positions discussed in detail in the ancient writings. They range from the simplest and most basic to the downright adventurous. First, let us look at some of the more basic sexual positions as put forth in the Kama Sutra:

Blossoming. The Kama Sutra calls this the Utphallaka, and the position may remind someone of a cross between the popular missionary position and a Pilates bridge pose. In the blossoming position, the woman raises her vagina at a level over her head, and the man enters her missionary-style. This position is particularly helpful for couples where the woman has a smaller vagina relative to a larger penis for the man. The blossoming position is also a great workout for the female's core.

In the blossoming position, both the man and the woman see each other's bodies and facial expressions in full view, basking in each other's naked glory. The woman gets to enjoy her own pleasure while also taking in the sight of her partner thrusting and enjoying her nether region. The man, on the other hand, will enjoy the sight of her face revelling in pleasure, her body responding to his movements, and her breasts bouncing in rhythm to his thrusts. As such, although the utphallaka position is not as close in proximity between two lovers, it is highly erotic.

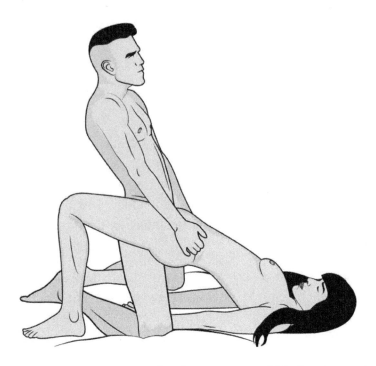

Envelopment. This position, also known as veshititaka, is particularly helpful for couples where the woman has a larger vagina and the man has a smaller penis. In envelopment, the woman will cross her legs as she is being penetrated, thus closing in around his member and allowing for more friction. Crossing the legs will make the entrance to the female vagina smaller, thus wrapping more tightly around the penis. During intercourse, the man will feel more pleasure because of the smaller orifice, while the woman's vaginal walls will also experience more friction.

In veshititaka, the woman may also practice clenching her muscles around the penis during penetration, which adds to the envelopment around his penis and increases the sensations for both partners. The position frees up the woman's hands to caress the man's buttocks or back, while the man can also stimulate her breasts, neck, or thighs.

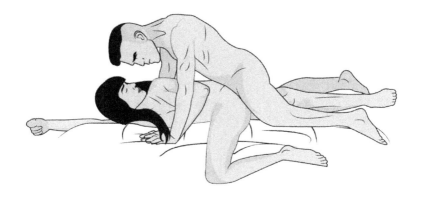

Expanding. This position is the opposite of envelopment. Called vijirimbhitaka in the Kama Sutra, expanding pertains to the woman raising one-leg during intercourse, similar to yoga leg lifts. The movement allows more of the penis to enter the vagina and is suggested to couples where the man has a larger member. In the expanding position, the woman lets the man fill her inner sanctum by opening more of her orifice to him. This position should be done gently at first, allowing the woman's member to adjust to the penis size, as the man slowly enters. More lubrication would be needed to make penetration easier especially if size is an issue.

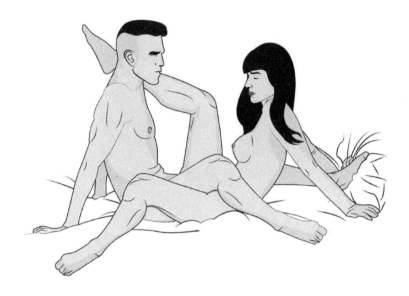

Impalement. Known in the Kama Sutra as shulachitaka, this position refers to the woman placing one foot on the man's head and submitting to penetration. It looks and sounds difficult but is quite easy to achieve especially for couples who are into erotic explorations.

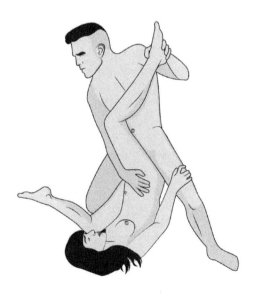

Lotus. This is akin to the lotus position in yoga, where the woman sits in a lotus position and then allows the man to enter her from the front. It does require some flexibility but is quite easy to achieve. The lotus position is great for couples who want to try sexual techniques that allow for face-to-face intercourse and lots of eye contact, but also need the increased penetration depth allowed by the lotus position.

The lotus position is ideal no matter the size difference between the man and the woman, as neither partner must worry about having to support the other person's weight. Both partners will have their hands free to stroke each other's hair, face, back, thighs, buttocks, and other areas. Also, in this technique the female's clitoris is easily accessible for manual stimulation, increasing female sensation.

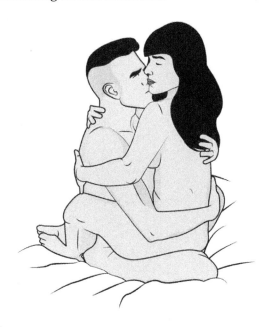

The Cow. In today's colloquial terms, this is now known as the doggy-style position. The cow, or dhenuka in the Kama Sutra, pertains to the man mounting the woman from behind as she is in mid-plank position. Many men consider this among the most pleasurable positions for them because of the angle of penetration. For the woman, the cow position also increases stimulation of the vagina because it allows for deeper penetration, and the man can also thrust in circular motions to increase the sensations. The woman may also reach under and caress her partner's scrotum during penetration.

This position is particularly popular because it allows either the man or the woman to stimulate the clitoris during penetration. As the speed and depth of the penetration increases, stimulation may be timed with the thrusts, inducing female climax. The man's hands can hold on to the woman's hair, shoulders, waist, or hips for deeper thrusts, or simply caress these erogenous zones for increased sensation. Many men also admit that they like the way their female partner looks from this angle, where the buttocks are in full view, the breasts hang low and bounce with the rhythm, and the woman's back moves with his thrusts.

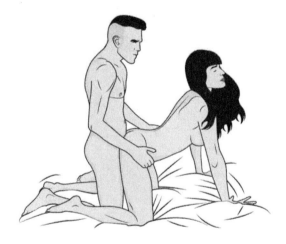

City Dweller. This position is big on eye-to-eye contact between the two partners. The woman will sit on the man's lap, facing him, wrapping her legs around his body, and then inserts the penis into her vagina. This very erotic and intimate position allows for a lot of caressing and clitoral stimulation. As the man penetrates the woman, he can use one hand to stimulate her clitoris, moving the other hand to cup her back or buttocks for deeper thrusts. In the city dweller position, the woman has control of the speed and intensity of the penetration, so she can focus on her pleasure and guide the man's penis into her nether region where she can feel the most stimulation.

The city dweller position is ideal for couples where the woman has a smaller vagina and wants penetration to be slower and gentler at first. To increase her arousal and ease the penetration, the man may also kiss or lick her ears, neck, nape, shoulders, or nipples, or they may engage in heavy kissing. As the vagina relaxes, more of the penis may be inserted, gradually until it is fully inside her member. She can then control the tempo until she reaches her climax.

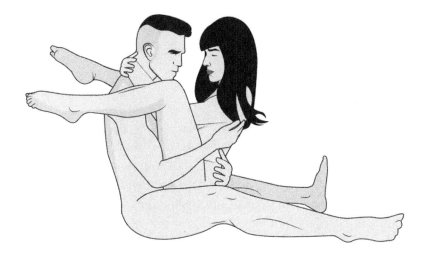

Lateral Box. This very simple sexual position involves the partners lying on their sides, facing each other, and their genitals touching each other. Slowly, the man inserts the penis into her vagina as they lie side by side, his hand guiding her closer to him. Kama Sutra calls this the parshva samputa. This position is great for partners who do not want their partner to have to support their weight, if they want to be able to kiss deeply during intercourse, or if either partner enjoys cupping the other person's buttocks during sex.

Many couples enjoy this position because it is not as physically strenuous. If you have both had a long day or just want to relax after a long time of travel but would still like to enjoy a hot bout of lovemaking, the lateral box is very laid-back and intimate. The tempo does not have to be rushed, and you can draw it out if you want, taking your time to enjoy the feeling of being connected physically while looking at each other and relishing the emotional bond.

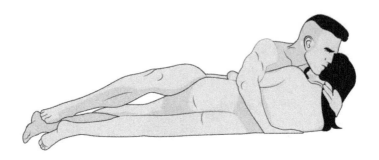

Closed Box. A variation of the style above, the closed box position or uttana samputa is done with the woman lying down, limbs stretched out, as the man is on top, pressing into her hips and penetrating from between the thighs. Again, just as the previous sexual position, the closed box is laid back and not as physically demanding, so it is great for partners who are feeling quite amorous at the end of a tiring day. Sexual intercourse can still be achieved but in a more relaxed and slow tempo.

One benefit of the closed box position is it allows the man to use his free hand to reach around and directly stimulate his partner's clitoris while he is penetrating from behind. Also, women who enjoy being kissed in the ears, nape, neck, or shoulders during sex will enjoy this position. The closed box leaves these erogenous zones free for the man to nibble on while he is inside her.

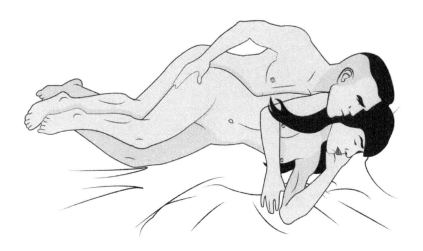

Frontal Box. Another variation of the box style is the frontal box. This time around, the woman has her knees folded up against her breasts as the man is penetrating from a doubled-up position in front of her. This position is suggested for men with large penises. In this variation, the form of the woman with her knees up against her breasts opens more of her orifice to his member. The angle will make it easier for a larger penis to then slowly penetrate, with the woman holding him and guiding the insertion.

In the frontal box position, the man also has access to the woman's lower back and buttocks, allowing him to caress or lightly spank these areas during penetration. Meanwhile, the woman can stroke his hair, face, or shoulders, or hold on to his torso as he penetrates. She can also reach inside and stimulate her clitoris as he is inside her vagina until she reaches her release.

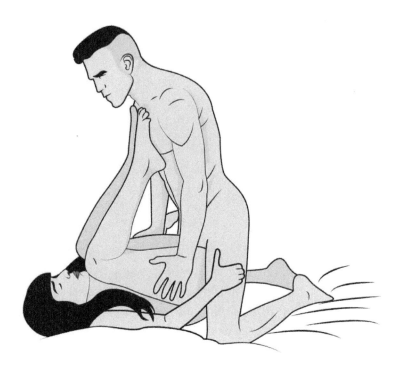

Bent. Called bhagnaka in the Kama Sutra, the bent position requires the woman to raise her thighs, her arms clasped over them and in locked position, as the man grips her and penetrates. Simple, but very sexually stimulating for both, this is one of the more popular of the basic Kama Sutra sex positions. In the bent position, a deeper penetration is achieved as the woman's pelvis is elevated, while the man's pelvic movements stimulate her clitoris. With the woman's arms clasped over her thighs, she can also hold on to his buttocks or torso during penetration.

Women who like deep penetration from their partner enjoy the bent position as it opens more of her orifice to his longer, deeper thrusts. At the same time, the man also has greater access to her clitoris and can stimulate it while penetrating her, increasing sensations for both. As the

140

vagina secretes more lubrication, the penis slides in and out of the orifice with more ease.

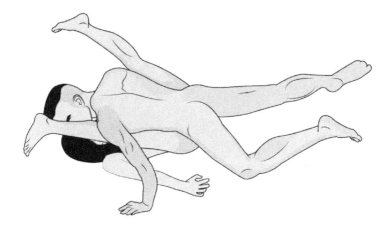

As you try these different Kama Sutra sex positions, remember to keep an open line of communication and ask your partner how he or she feels about each style. Humans are wired differently, and some biological and physical considerations and factors also have their effect on sexual stimulation and pleasure, so being open about what you both like and don't like will help you achieve that sexual nirvana together.

It would be helpful to have lubricating products handy during your lovemaking. Lubrication products such as petroleum jelly help make penetration easier for the woman especially for couples who contend with a smaller vagina size for her, or a larger penis size for him. Aside from lube products, sex toys such as dildos or vibrators of varying sizes may help her vagina relax before penetration, while also adding a bit of variety and imagination to the lovemaking session.

Now, are you ready to try some of the more adventurous positions as laid out in the Kama Sutra? In the next chapter, let us investigate the more acrobatic, challenging, and sexually-charged positions you and your lover may want to test tonight.

Chapter Summary

- Some of the basic sexual positions in the Kama Sutra mirror poses in yoga and Pilates, requiring basic flexibility and core strength.
- There are beginner sex positions for different considerations, such as penis and vagina sizes.
- In these poses, communication is important for the couple to maintain. What works for some couples may not be as pleasurable for others.

Chapter Seven: Advanced Kama Sutra Sex Positions

The sex life of couples can become quite monotonous and boring after a while if the same positions, activities, and styles are repeated over and over again. Thankfully, there are ways to spice things up in the bedroom and reinject life and passion into the relationship. The sections of the Kama Sutra detailing sexual techniques are particularly explicit about various positions that may appear to be more adventurous and challenging than the usual. These more advanced positions may be just the right ingredients needed to heat up your nights once again and rekindle that passion.

Before trying out any of the advanced Kama Sutra techniques, remember to keep the safety of yourself and your partner at the top of the considerations. Are you and your partner in generally healthy condition, and physically able to perform such actions? How safe is your environment? Are there potentially hazardous items such as furniture or lighting fixtures within the vicinity that may pose dangers if unintentionally toppled over or hit during lovemaking?

Of course, the comfort level of both parties should always be prioritized. Be sure to talk openly about what you both would like to try and set clear guidelines as to how far your sexual adventures would go. When parameters are set, stick to them and do not be afraid to voice out any concerns you may have about certain techniques you may not feel entirely comfortable trying.

The following are some of the more advanced sexual positions taught in the writings of the Kama Sutra:

Erotic V. For couples with that acrobatic flair, this is a must-try. The erotic V involves the woman sitting down on the edge of a table, with the man standing in front of her, bending his legs as he enters her. Then, the woman puts her arms back, leaning on the bed or table while wrapping her legs around his waist, as he then leans back and begins thrusting into her. Balance is the key in this position, so make sure you are both quite flexible (and the table is sturdy).

In the erotic V position, the woman is on top, but the man is in charge of the speed and depth of the penetration. She can cup his face, arms, torso, or buttocks during intercourse, while he can tilt her head using his hand, or grab her waist or buttocks for additional thrust. Kissing and necking are very much possible in this technique, and the angle allows for deeper penetration and greater stimulation for both the penis and the vagina.

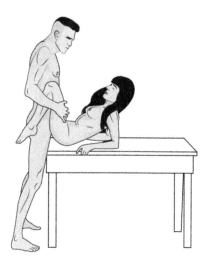

Fantastic Rocking Horse. For women who like to be on top, this position can be very pleasurable. The man will sit cross-legged and lean back, supported by his arms. The woman will then kneel over his lap, her thighs wrapped around his lower body, as she inserts the penis into her vagina. In this position, the woman has total control over the speed and the penetration. If the position is a bit difficult for the man to maintain his balance, the fantastic rocking horse can be done against a wall or bedpost.

For the woman, core strength and lower back stability are essential for maximum pleasure from this position. The fantastic rocking horse, meanwhile, is great exercise for the man's upper body and arms. Kissing, petting, and necking can be easily done in this position because the lovers are face-to-face. The man can stimulate the woman's clitoris as she guides the rhythmic movement, and use another hand to caress her nape, back, buttocks, or breasts. She, on the other hand, can use his shoulders to balance herself and help in the up-and-down movements.

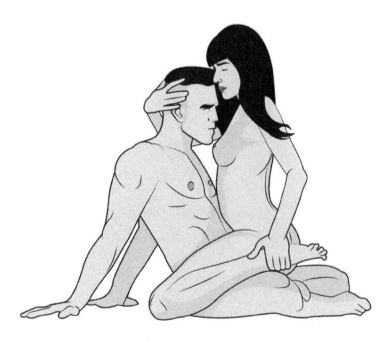

Catherine Wheel. Couples who are in excellent physical shape can try this position which is a bit more complicated than it looks. The partners sit opposite each other, face to face, then the woman wraps her legs around the man's torso. He penetrates her, wrapping one leg over the woman to keep her in position, while she braces with her hands. The man controls the movement using his torso, with his elbows supporting

146

both their weight. It's a sexual position but can also feel like an upper body workout for the man.

This position has some similarities with the fantastic rocking horse, but differs with his leg keeping her in place, and with the man doing the movement. Couples where the man is larger in size and the woman is lighter or more petite will find this position very enjoyable. The vertical thrusting inside the vagina is particularly pleasurable for the male partner, while the woman can focus on her pleasure without worrying about supporting her own weight, or his. Their hands are also free to caress each other or stimulate the clitoris during penetration.

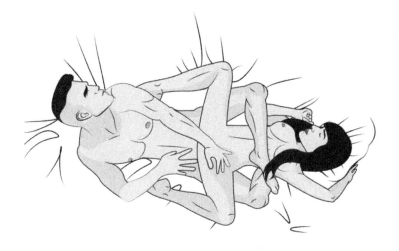

The Ape (Reverse Cowgirl) The Ape position is achieved with the man on his back. Then, the woman sits down, facing backwards, sliding his penis into her vagina as she keeps herself propped up on his legs. This very sensual position requires a lot of balance and coordination between the partners. If the woman is strong in the legs she can stand on her feet and squat into this position, controlling the movements while the male can rest so he has more energy for the next position.

Once this style is achieved, the unique angle will be intensely pleasurable for both partners. It is a different angle from many other positions in the bedroom and the male partner may find his manhood exploring new crevices in her special place he never thought existed. The woman will enjoy the stimulation in areas of her vagina not normally reached during intercourse.

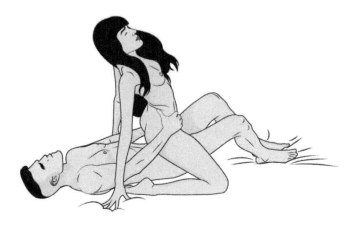

Ascent to Desire. For men who can lift their partner's weight easily, this position can be tried. The man stands with hips apart, knees bent slightly. He lifts the woman onto him, and as she wraps her legs around his hips, he enters her. In this position, the woman is in control of the penetration as the man supports her weight.

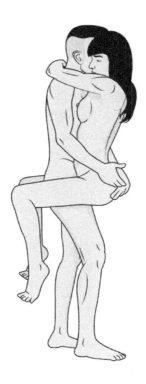

This position requires the man to be able to carry the woman's weight with his arms, back, and upper body. It is a great position for couples with bigger males and smaller females to try. The position allows for deeper vaginal penetration which increases the sensory excitement for both partners, while the clitoris of the female rubs against the male's pelvis and lower stomach, intensifying the pleasure. In ascent to desire, the man's hands may be solely holding on to her buttocks or thighs for support, but the woman is free to use her hands to roam his body. Kissing and necking are also ideal for this position.

The Bridge. This position is quite challenging and only suitable if the man is very flexible and strong. He will make a bridge with his body as the woman straddles him, lowering herself onto his penis while keeping her weight on her feet. The woman then proceeds to move up and down to control the thrusting. This position is great for couples where one or both partners have had some gymnastics or aerobics experience, or are active in yoga or Pilates, both of which deal with stability and flexibility and have poses very similar to the bridge.

In this style, the woman is completely in control of the speed, intensity, and depth of the vaginal penetration, while the man must support his weight with his arms, so no direct stimulation of the female clitoris or other body parts may be performed. The woman, however, is free to pleasure her own clitoris, breasts, or other erogenous zones while she is moving up and down on his penis. Couples should be careful not to do this position for very extended periods of time, as the blood flow to the man's head may get to be too much.

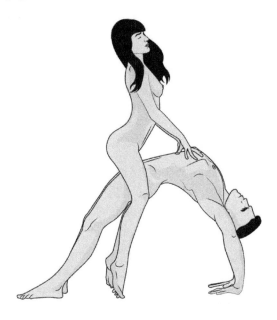

Double Decker. For small women and larger men, this position should be tried. With the man lying on his back, the woman sits on top of him, both facing the same direction. She leans back, propped up on her elbows, with her back against his chest. The man keeps her steady by holding her at the waist, penetrating at this angle.

The double decker sexual technique allows the woman to guide the man to those parts of her inner sanctum where she feels the most pleasure when penetrated. She can control the speed, angle, and depth, even moving back and forth or in circular motions to feel the full girth of his member in her nether region. The man, on the other hand, will particularly enjoy the vertical movement of her vagina on his manhood. The woman is free to also stimulate his scrotum with one hand while she is moving on top of him, while the man can use one hand to reach around and stimulate her clitoris and bring her to full sexual release.

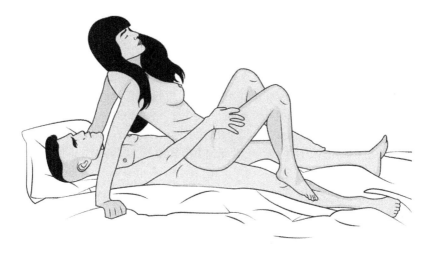

The Seduction. Women who have tried yoga may find this quite easy to master. She kneels and then leans back, with her ankles under her buttocks, then raises her arms above her head. The man kneels over her and penetrates from a planked position, keeping his weight on his forearms, thrusting into her deeply. In this technique, the woman opens more of her vagina to the man's penis, allowing him to probe deeper into every nook and cranny of her body. The arms raised over her head denotes complete surrender to his domination and the sexual pleasure that will follow.

In the seduction position, the man is free to control the speed, depth, and intensity of the penetration while looking into the eyes of his lover and watching her facial expressions as his manhood stimulates her inner sanctum. He may commence kissing, necking, or petting the woman

151

while penetrating her, and she can also guide him deeper into her by occasionally grabbing his torso or buttocks and pulling him closer.

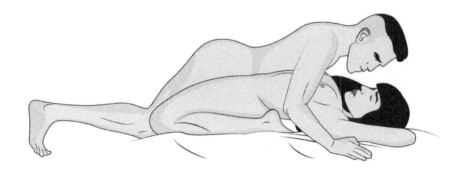

Crouching Tiger. The Crouching Tiger position allows the woman to stimulate her clitoris or his scrotum during penetration which makes this is an intensely pleasurable position to try. The man will lie back on the bed, his feet on the ground, and his hands holding up the woman's buttocks. The woman squats facing away from him, then lowers her vagina onto his penis. The woman controls the up and down movement while his hands help to support her weight.

This position has many similarities to the cow or doggy-style position, especially in the sensations as well as the angle of the penetration. The difference, however is the man is lying back in this technique, while the woman commences penetration by lowering herself into his manhood. Also, the woman takes charge of the rhythm and tempo of penetration in this intercourse technique. Couples who enjoy doing it doggy-style but would like to add a bit of variety to the position may try the crouching tiger. This sex position, aside from being very pleasurable for both partners, is a great leg and back workout for the female. It also allows the man to enjoy the naked glory of the woman from behind as he basks in the view of his partner taking him in and riding his member.

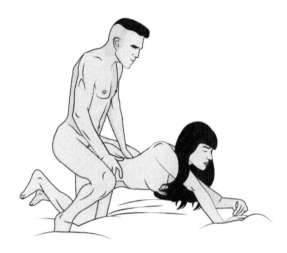

Broken Flute. This position is also called the venudaritaka and is among the most bizarre in the Kama Sutra. The woman lies down, puts her foot on the man's shoulder, then takes it off and puts the other foot on his other shoulder, all while he is inside her. It does require good core and leg strength, but the Broken Flute position is one you should try if you want something new.

In the broker flute technique, the movement of the woman's legs being alternately placed on the man's shoulders will cause her vagina to contract, expand, and caress his erection while inside her, causing an altogether different sensation. The movement also allows her to discover new areas of her vagina that need to be pleasured during penetration. The man will enjoy the sight of his partner taking in his erection and making it her own pleasure object, and during penetration the man can also freely roam the length of her body, even stimulating her clitoris which will be easily accessible in this position.

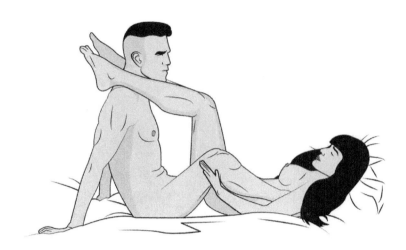

The Spin. In the Kama Sutra, this is the paravrittaka, where the woman is seated on top of the man during penetration, and then spins around 180 degrees. This is quite difficult for the woman to master but is intensely pleasurable for the man and the woman. The sensations felt in this circular motion are unlike any other sensations felt in other sexual positions, and there is also the rush of adrenaline due to the more physical nature of this technique, especially for the female.

Some women may find the spinning motion to be uncomfortable or cause a bit of nausea, so it is advised to go slowly at first, with the man providing as much support and balance as possible. The spin is one of the more adventurous and strenuous of the advanced Kama Sutra positions, but don't knock it before you have tried it. You just might find a different head rush when performing this position. For the man, be generous with kisses, caresses, and stimulation to her various erogenous zones before, during, and after the spin position to make the experience more pleasurable.

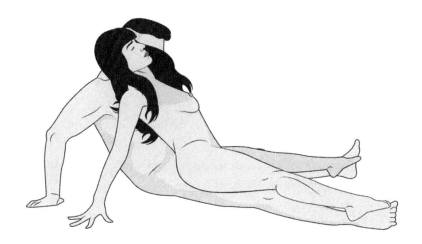

As you can see, many of these advanced sexual positions from the Kama Sutra will test your stamina, flexibility, balance, coordination, or all of these (among other skills). They may be hard to achieve at first, but once you master these positions, you will find your sex life to be more varied and adventurous. There are, of course, more positions detailed in the texts of the Kama Sutra which you can also explore as you become more of an expert in these styles.

Chapter Summary

- New and unique sex positions play a role in revitalizing a relationship that has become monotonous.
- Before trying the more challenging Kama Sutra positions, ensure that you are physically fit to handle them.
- Discuss with your partner first regarding your level of comfort. When in doubt, don't.
- Some of the advanced sexual positions in the Kama Sutra allow the woman to be on top and in control of the penetration depth and speed.
- For advanced sexual positions, the man must remember to also use his hands to stimulate the woman's clitoris, breasts, and other erogenous zones during penetration.

Final Words

Sex should be viewed as a healthy and normal part of your relationship with your partner. The level of intimacy and compatibility you reach with your significant other is undeniably tied to your sexual relationship. When there is conflict or unresolved tension, sex is often one of those activities that tends to fall by the wayside because it requires a level of closeness and emotional connection unlike any other activity. Likewise, a healthy relationship also often translates to an open and vibrant sex life.

It is true that sex is not all there is to a romantic relationship, but it cannot be denied that it does play a major part in the dynamics of the partnership. As human beings, our sexuality is part of who we are. It is wired into our thinking and plays a big role in much of our daily thinking and decision making, whether we are aware of it or not. Because of this fact, it is important to maintain a balanced, well-rounded view of sexuality in general if true happiness and satisfaction in life is to be achieved.

The beauty of the Kama Sutra is the unashamed way it ties together various sexual topics into its other lessons on life and the pursuit of happiness. That is why, even in this modern age, the tenets of the Kama Sutra continue to be used and studied by people all over the world looking to enhance their lovemaking prowess. While not necessarily an exclusive sex manual, the Kama Sutra has become known as the standard by which most other depictions of human sexuality and behavior are measured against.

How should these learnings affect you in a positive and enriching way? Hopefully, as you become familiar with the Kama Sutra through the pages of this book, you become more attuned to your sexual skills and the needs of your partner and develop a path towards achieving that peak of sexual pleasure together. Sexual intimacy is more than just an orgasm at the end of the act of lovemaking. Intimacy encompasses daily life and brings the couple together, allowing them to see the world differently and with the same perspective.

Through the ancient writings of the Kama Sutra, the hope is that you will enhance your skills as a lover, with the focus not on your personal gratification but on pleasuring your significant other, keeping his or her physical needs ahead of yours. The mastery of the techniques of the Kama Sutra should bring out that amazing and unforgettable lover in you. Through these techniques, you can reignite the fires of desire and connect with your partner sexually as if it were your first time all over again.

The Kama Sutra, with its valuable lessons on life, happiness, sexuality, and the human experience, continues to transcend generations and appeal to enthusiasts regardless of what era in human history they may come from. Hopefully, through the concepts of lovemaking portrayed in the Kama Sutra, you will begin to see sex as an art, requiring attention to detail and constant analysis of one's skills in order to produce a masterpiece.

By now you should have a huge understanding of Kama Sutra and the techniques & positions needed in order to reach the climax of your partner. If you found this book helpful please leave a positive review on Amazon as it is greatly appreciated and keeps me being able to deliver high quality books.

Tantric Sex

Master The Art Of Tantric Sex
Through Love Connecting Guided Sex
Positions And Techniques, With
Pictures

Max Bush

Table Of Contents

Introduction

You may have heard of Tantra. Tantra is a system of ideas derived from ancient Hindu and Buddhist traditions and practices. But what about Tantric Sex? Tantric belief systems see sex and eroticism as being natural aspects of life; furthermore, sex is viewed as a path to spirituality. The Tantric view of sexuality is unabashed. Some aspects of Tantric Sex have been perceived as extreme, however they are not commonplace. This book will focus on introducing you, the reader, to the ideas behind Tantric Sex and provide a practical guide on how to incorporate Tantric Sex in your sex life.

You are probably thinking to yourself, *okay, what is the difference between sex and Tantric Sex?* Sex is often reduced to a simple, mechanical act. But we know it is, and *should* be, more than a simple, mechanical act. You want your sex life to be open; you want your sex life to help you understand yourself and your partner. Opening yourself to the Tantric practice will help you with exactly that!

But maybe you are still thinking: I do not know what Tantra is and how it plays into sexuality. Well, let's dive right in!

First, one must understand the openness of sexuality. Sexuality has oddly been a contentious issue. Sexuality is a normal part of life for most individuals, yet an embarrassment toward sexuality has existed for centuries. In recent times however, we have seen an openness toward sexuality and an understanding of sexuality's breadth. Tantric Sex is not stringent, but it does require one thing from a participant: an openness. This does not mean you need to follow everything or do something that makes you uncomfortable; rather, you should keep an open mind in your approach to sexuality.

Tantric Sex is meant for you to emancipate yourself from any boundaries. Tantric Sex believes you will reach the Divine through sexuality. Sexuality and Sexual Thought is accepted and is seen as an important facet of life in the Tantra philosophy. As mentioned above, Tantric Sex is not stringent. It is not a set of ideas that must be followed. You do not have to declare that you engage in Tantric Sex or join a group that shares your ideas. Everyone's Tantric Sex experiences and perceptions will be different. No one is more or less 'Tantric' than you are due to their perspective on Tantric Sex. Ask a hundred people about Tantric Sex and you will receive a hundred explanations as to what it is. Like the openness of the Tantra philosophy itself, the experience of Tantric Sex is also open.

There are certain sexual acts which have been popular amongst Tantric Sex practitioners. This book will provide some of these sexual acts which should help you begin your journey with Tantric Sex. These acts will also help you gain a grounding of Tantric Sex as you continue your journey and open yourself to new experiences.

As this book is intended to be a guide I would suggest you refer to it whenever possible. To ensure that Tantra remains a consistent approach to your sex life, you want to use this book as a guide which can be revisited at any time. Tantra is not a goal to achieve and as a result, there is no destination. For making the most out of this book and ensuring you follow through with the lessons provided, I would recommend keeping a notebook and pen by your side as you read. You will be referring to this notebook to practice the exercises, recording any progress, and keeping a schedule or planning ahead for the exercises. This may seem like homework, but it will ensure that you are able to make the most out of your learning about Tantric Sex and apply it to your sex life. The first chapter focuses on individual exercises, though I would recommend you have your partner read it when you are finished. If they follow the exercises and record their reflections as you do, you will both receive the great benefits of Tantric Sex together!

Tantric Sex and Tantra in general, is known to utilize factors like chakras and energy which you may or may not be familiar with. Many individuals are intimidated by Tantric Sex because they feel they need a deep understanding of a variety of topics beforehand, ranging from metaphysics, to Hindu traditions and rituals, to chakras and energy. But do not worry! This book is focused on applying Tantric traditions and practices for the modern reader. Regardless of what knowledge you may or may not have about Tantra, this book will give practices which are straightforward; an understanding of the importance of these practices and how they will benefit your sex life will be provided.

Before moving on, take a moment to reflect upon your sex life and your sexuality so far. Take out your notebook and pen and answer the following questions. Answer in as much detail as possible:

1. What was the attitude toward sexuality as you were growing up? Did you grow up in a household that had a liberal or conservative attitude toward sexuality? Or do you not know because it was never discussed?
2. What was *your* attitude toward sexuality as you were growing up?
3. What was the prevailing attitude toward sexuality in the society you lived in? Has it changed? If you live in a different society, how does it differ with your previous society?
4. If you could change other person's attitudes toward sexuality what would you do?
5. What are your current attitudes toward sexuality? Are you happy with this? Do you want to change anything about your perspective?
6. Do you experiment often with your sexuality and your sex life? Do you try new things? Do you engage in much foreplay? Do you set scenes or use toys or props?
7. What do you feel about your partner? Do you feel your partner has a healthy attitude toward sexuality? Do you wish to change anything about your partner's sexuality or their approach to sex? If you do not have a partner, describe what you would like in an ideal partner.

8. What do you think your partner feels about you and your approach to sexuality? How would you like your ideal partner to view your approach to sexuality?
9. What would you like your partner to think of who you are as a person? If you do not have a partner how would you want them to perceive you?
10. Finally, what do you already know about Tantric Sex and what are your thoughts on what you expect before moving on to the further exercises in this book?

Chapter One: Solo Tantra

In this chapter, you will learn how to prepare yourself for Tantric Sex.

You have answered quite a few questions and are now ready to explore the world of Tantric Sex! You will hopefully have dispelled any apprehension you may have toward Tantric Sex and are ready to open yourself up to experimentation and discovery. Since this book is about bringing Tantric Sex to your relationship, *you* are not the only one who must open up to embrace Tantric Sex. However, before you begin to discuss Tantric Sex with your partner, you must first open *yourself* up and make *yourself* comfortable with the practices.

This first chapter will focus on creating an atmosphere within yourself that will be conducive to Tantric Sex. Ensure that you develop a discipline with the following practices in this chapter; you will need to change your attitude toward sexuality, and therefore alter your lifestyle in order to receive the benefits of Tantric Sex. Now that you have that in mind, it is time to jump right in!

Take A Breather!

One practice essential to Tantric Sex is something you are doing as you are reading this book: breathing. Breathing is something we do all the time, and therefore we do not realize its importance; we also seldom breathe consciously. You may not realize it now, but breathing will play a huge part in improving your Tantric Sex techniques with your partner. But for now, you must master breathing for yourself.

Pause for a moment and follow these exercises to improve your breathing techniques:

1. If possible, find a quiet space where you can be isolated from others and from distractions. You may sit or stand straight. Ensure that your back is as erect as can be. Now, breathe in deeply and let your breath flow outwards by opening your mouth and breathing out heavily. Repeat this for at least five minutes.

2. Our politeness causes us to be embarrassed about yawning. But yawning is a great way of breathing out and improving our breathing techniques. Perhaps you will still want to cover your mouth or restrain yourself in public. But in your private space, practice yawning – it will have the same effect as the heavy breathing in and out.

3. Breathe and moan. This is something you probably already do during any form of sexual activity. But otherwise you would not think about breathing and moaning to your fullest extent. That would be awkward, would it not? Well, you are following Tantric Sex, and nothing is awkward! Once again, make sure you are standing or seated and have your back as erect as possible; Take in your deep breaths and hold them in for as long as you can. When you exhale moan as loudly and with as much fervor as you can. Repeat this for at least five minutes.

The above exercises should help you develop a discipline of breathing. This will serve as a solid grounding for opening yourself up for Tantric Sex and Sexual exploration of yourself and your partner. Next, we will do a silent activity: meditating!

Meditation

Meditation is very popular but is often misunderstood. This book focuses on Tantric Sex for the modern world, so Meditation will not be defined by its stereotype: that you must sit with your legs crossed, close your eyes, imagine light flowing through your body and chanting in Sanskrit. You are welcome to practice this form of Meditation of course; but, just as there are no hard and fast rules with Tantric Sex, you must understand that the same applies to Meditation.

What is the purpose of Meditation? The goal of Meditation is for one to relax one's mind. I am willing to bet that your life is hectic. The modern world presents us with many distractions and we must find a way to relax our mind and bodies. This form of relaxation is Meditation. For the purposes of this book, I want you to take a moment and reflect on what is your preferred way to meditate. Find time out of your week to practice this Meditation and be disciplined about it. If you wish to lie on your bed with your eyes closed, do so, but ensure that you can do it on all or most days of the week. If going for a run is your preferred method for Meditation, then ensure you are disciplined about going for a run and are disciplined about your run!

Laugh

Have you ever laughed during sex? Despite the absurdity of the question, I assure you it is entirely serious! Maybe you did and were embarrassed, and your partner was taken aback. Or maybe you would consider it strange if such an incident occurred during sexual activity. Well, you know the pattern by now: Tantric Sex wants you to dispel such ridiculous notions. Just as you would smile during moments of sexual gratification, why would you not laugh? Laughter is the ultimate expression of bliss; a laugh is far more expressive than a smile. Just as you have practiced your breathing and meditating techniques, you must also practice laughing!

Find your quiet space and practice these exercises:

1. Laugh out loud! Breath in deeply and let out your breath in loud, unabashed bursts of laughter. Repeat this for at least five minutes.
2. Engage in more activities that make you laugh. Whether it is reading a comic novel or watching a stand-up comedy special, fill your life with more laughter.
3. In moments of distress, laugh at the situation to relax yourself. This may not always be possible and is challenging based on the situation – but give it your best shot!
4. When you smile, laugh. As I stated before, laughing is far more expressive than smiling. So, turn that smile into a laugh whenever you can! Even a chuckle will suffice!

Focus!

The final step is to improve your focus. This is perhaps the most difficult step, but it will make you a more focused individual. Take a moment to think about your partner or a partner whom you desire; can you accurately describe their features and personality? Take a sheet of paper from your notebook and jot down your answers to the following questions in as much detail as possible about this individual:

1. Describe in the detail, the eyes of the individual. Go beyond their color: are they a light brown or are they as dark as a starless night? Are they large or small? Are they expressive or unassuming? What about around their eyes?

170

2. Describe their physique. Do not focus on if they are slim, average build, or heavyset. Do they have wide hips? Long legs? A puffed chest? Broad shoulders?
3. Describe their personality. Does this individual have a relaxed approach? Are they anxious? Are they reticent or boisterous?
4. What attracts you to this person? It can range from their career to how well they tell a joke. Be free for this one, remembering to be as descriptive as possible.
5. Once you have answered the above four questions in as much detail as possible, you can revisit them at a later time to add additional information/observations if you feel you can. You can also now have free reign in whatever else you wish to write about this individual. This can range from habits or characteristics they have which arouse you, to sexual fantasies you have about them, to their taste in anything from food to films. The sky is the limit; your goal should be to have an understanding on who the person is. The more detail you can provide should be an indication of how focused you are on them and who they are as an individual.

You may wonder what these particular exercises are for. Remember that Tantric Sex is considered sacred. It is intended to be focused and conscious and not a simple, mechanical act. Being able to focus on your partner and understand them beforehand will help you when engaging in Tantric Sex with them.

Before we move on, you must ensure you set a discipline of practicing the exercises in this chapter, so you have a sufficient grounding for when you move on to practices with your partner.

Turn to a blank page in your notebook; you will be creating a schedule or planner to set time aside from your week to practice the aforementioned exercises. It does not have to be fancy, you can organize your calendar as you see fit but it should follow this example:

Monday - Friday

10 AM to 10:30 AM – Breathing Exercises

12 PM to 12:30 PM – Laughing Exercises

4 PM to 4:30 PM – Meditation

9 PM to 9:30 PM – Writing (Focus Exercises)

You want to ensure you stick to your schedule as consistently as possible to guarantee you get the most benefit from these exercises.

On another blank page in your notebook, you will be keeping a Progress Log. With the Progress Log you will keep track of what you have learned and gained so far from the exercises. The goal is to observe what you are feeling from the exercises. As there is no 'right or wrong' with Tantric Sex, there are no right or wrong answers from these exercises. Here is how you can format your Progress Log:

Write the date at the top of the page. Write each of the questions below and leave a few spaces between questions to fill in your answers. Here are the questions to answer:

1. How do you feel after completing your Breathing Exercises?
2. How do you feel after completing your Laughing Exercises?
3. How do you feel after completing your Meditation?
4. Do you feel your focus on your partner or desired partner has improved since writing about their features?

Ideally you will answer these questions in as much detail as possible and each Progress Log will open a new avenue of expression. At the end of each month, take the time to read through your Progress Logs to reflect on how you have improved with your exercises and what you have learned. Ideally, each time you log your progress there will be something new.

The preceding exercises are not strictly of a sexual nature. But as I mentioned, they are essential for opening yourself up for later practices. There are more practices one can do individually at any time to prepare themselves for a sexual experience or to simply become more 'sexual' as an individual. One must always keep in mind that Tantric Sex is an unabashed attitude toward sex. I promised I would not overwhelm you with any historical perspective, but it is crucial to remember than as a tradition steeped in Hindu philosophy, sexuality is seen as a natural part of life and therefore, cultivating a healthy sexual appetite is normal and not something to be embarrassed about.

Going Solo

At any time, one should feel free to stimulate and awaken their sexual energy, whether they are planning to have sex soon or in the future – or not at all! If you decide to incorporate Tantric Sex into your life, you must be sexual. I will now introduce you to some practices which are more sexual in nature in comparison to the previous practices.

Here are a variety of practices which fall under the umbrella of self-loving or Solo Tantra, if you like:

1. Masturbation: you are welcome and encouraged to love yourself and try to provide yourself with as much sexual pleasure as you can.
2. Dressing and undressing: what clothing makes you feel sexually awakened? Is it a particular costume, lingerie, or nothing at all? You do not have to exclusively be in this state of dress or undress when you are with your partner. Feel unabashed and parade around your home and check yourself out in your mirror in the clothing (or lack of) that increases your sexual energy.

3. You are never too old to play with toys: vibrators, dildos, pocket pussies, self-flagellators, blow-up dolls etc., are all welcome for you to use.
4. Dancing: giving a lap dance to your partner is always fun as is receiving one; you can use your free time to practice a lap dance or pole dance or any form of seductive and sexual body expression.
5. Setting the scene: once you begin the Tantric Sex experience with your partner, you will learn more about environment and ambience. In the meantime, visualize your ideal setting for sex; for instance, if it is your bedroom how would you like the bedroom to look? Would you want flowers on the floor? Any particular blanket on the bed? Any music playing in the background? How will the bedroom be lit? Experiment with setting your environment to your liking. Play around with different ideas so you are ready to set the scene for your partner.

As you embark on your journey with Tantric Sex, you must be disciplined about awakening and stimulating your sexual energy. Your approach to sexuality should be as if you were adopting a lifestyle change. If you wanted to change your physique you would approach a discipline regarding your diet and exercise. Similarly, your approach to sexuality has to follow the same regimen. Dedicate your free time to pursuing the growth of your sexual energy; you should now see it as crucial to your life and your well-being as your diet and paying your bills are!

You would have noticed by now that the phrase 'sexual energy' has been tossed around. You are probably wondering what it means. Sexual Energy can be expressed as sexual desire, virility, passion, etc. To be enjoy sex and receive the benefits of Tantric Sex your sexual energy must be awakened at all times. This is something to cultivate and the discipline of the exercises you have learned so far will help in cultivating sexual energy.

Tantric Sex is not ashamed of the body and realizes its importance. The physical is important and any notion of separating yourself from your body should be dispelled. Your sexual energy is naturally present in your genitals, but Tantric Sex looks at the body in a holistic fashion – therefore, your entire body is an instrument for sexual activity. You will think of your genitals as sexual, but do you think of your hands as inherently sexual? You may be aroused by your partners breasts, genitals, and buttocks. When you kiss their lips, you think of their lips as sexual. But what about their nose? What about their knees?

Sexual Energy

Take a moment to pause and reflect. Are there any parts of the body (yours and/or your partners) which do *not* feel sexual to you? Do you not see them as inherently sexual? Have you not utilized them for sexual activity? Have you caressed your partners body with your fingers, but not your elbow? Give it a try and incorporate your elbow in your self-loving or Solo-Tantra exercises. Utilize as much of your body as you can to explore different facets of your sexuality.

Here are some practices you and your partner can follow (separately or together) to awaken the sexual energy in your body as a whole and train your endurance towards your sex life:

1. You have learned about focusing. Now, here is a challenging exercise to see how well you can focus with your eyes. Either stand erect or lie on your back and keep your eyes focused on one object or area of the space you are in. Remaining in a prone position, move your eyes as far back as you can; follow this with looking down at your toes. Pick parts of your body to observe with your eyes without altering your body's prone position; you can look

at your genitals, your arms, knees, nose etc. There are no restrictions!

2. You have used your mouth quite a lot so far. You have practiced your breathing and have even laughed out loud! I want you to continue to practice using your mouth to enhance sexual energy. How many sounds can you make with your mouth? Can you shriek? Can you make 'click' sounds? Can you roll your tongue around and produce a melodious tune? Can you whistle? Practice making sounds with your mouth. Practice and test the limits of your tongue as well: stick it out as far as you can. Move it around on the outside. Can you touch your nose and your chin with your tongue? If you flap your tongue up and down, how long would it take until you reach a stage of exhaustion? Give it a try and find out!

3. Other things to focus on your mouth are to ensure you have a strong jaw, strong (and clean!) teeth; is your mouth usually dry? What about your lips? Ensure that you are always properly hydrated. If you need to salivate do so – you want to ensure that your mouth and its' inner components are prepared for sexual activity.

4. How often do you move your head and neck during a sexual activity? From kissing to performing oral sex, our heads and necks are crucial for sexual activity – without us even realizing it! Some exercises you can do is to move your head and neck side to side and look up and down.

5. Next, we move on to the belly. Feel free to squeeze your belly, move it around and push in and out. Much of your energy comes from your belly and you want to ensure you feel relaxed in that area.

6. Finally, ensure that your torso and lower body is in order: a) thrust your pelvis back and forth b) shake your hips c) jump up and down d) bounce up and down on the balls of your feet.

Dance!

You may have noticed that the sixth point above replicates dancing. That is exactly what we will move on to next. Dancing makes an individuals' body agile and an agile body is crucial for sexual activity. The next set of practices will revolve all around dancing!

1. We will return to your hips and pelvis! Stretch your legs wide apart and shake your hips! Begin slowly and then speed things up to as rapid as you can tolerate; do this until you are exhausted with this particular movement – but be sure not to exhaust yourself completely!
2. Arch your back and stretch your pelvis as forward as possible.
3. Lean forward and push your buttocks out as far as possible.
4. Now, put your legs together and slowly swing your hips side to side.

Additional Exercises

The next step will come in handy later on. You will learn that Tantric Sex involves a lot of activities outside of intercourse; in order for these to offer gratification you want to ensure that you and your partner last as long as possible before finishing. This next exercise will help you discipline yourself for lasting longer.

Have you ever ejaculated before you wanted to? Ever tried to 'stop it' by tightening yourself? That is what this exercise is for:

1. Squeeze and tighten your genitals. Hold it for as long as you can without causing distress and then let go. Repeat for as often as you are comfortable.
2. Massage and tighten your genitals while massaging them; do this for as long as you are comfortable. Repeat for as often as you are comfortable.

You may associate Tantra with Yoga, which in turn you may associate with chanting. Tantric Sex also entails making noises to awaken your sexual energy. You have learned several techniques on utilizing your mouth to awaken your sexual energy. Here are some more exercises which are more detailed and precise:

1. Sit or stand with your back erect.
2. Slowly blow air out of your mouth with your lips rounded. Do this for as long as you can without exhausting yourself.
3. After a few minutes to catch your breath, repeat the above step, this time try to let out a soft hum as you blow out air.
4. Raise the sound of the hum and let the vibrations flow through your body.
5. Take a pause and catch your breath.

Repeat these above exercises with two other variations: firstly, by opening your mouth as wide as possible as opposed to rounded lips and secondly, by opening your lips but letting out the air and sounds through clenched teeth.

Finally, you need to be aware of what arouses you. I am sure you feel you already have the answers for this but if someone asks you, "What is your ultimate sexual fantasy?", how detailed and precise would you be in your answer? When you engage with your partner with Tantric Sex you will be setting a scene and catering your partners needs and desires, as they will for you. Before reaching that stage, you want to ensure that you have an understanding of yourself so that you can communicate effectively with your partner. With the below questions, feel free to test out the experiences to see what you enjoy.

Here are the things to consider and experiment with, beginning with the visuals:

1. What colors do you find erotic? Is there a particular color when applied to the interior design will set the mood for you? What color clothing on you or your partner will add the mood?
2. Is there a particular design aesthetic which attracts you? Do you like lingerie with a leopard print on it? Do you like a modern aesthetic or a rustic, antiquated look?
3. Do you like a room to be filled with light or dim? Do you prefer the natural light, light by an abundance of candles, or just by turning on the switch? Does the window need a particular view or no view at all?
4. Do you like a wide-open space or a confined space? Are you more aroused by a room where you and your partner can run around in or one where you are in close contact in every corner?

Next, think about what gives you aural pleasure:

1. What tone of voice arouses you? Do you like gentle whispering or boisterous oration?
2. What kind of words arouse you? Do you enjoy subtle romanticism, straightforwardness, or dirty talk? Are there particular words you like to be called? Remember, there is no shame in Tantric Sex, so do not hesitate to communicate to your partner what you like to be called.
3. What music and sounds do you enjoy?

Of course, the primary aspect of the sexual experience is the physical:

1. Where do you like being touched the most? What parts of your body bring you arousal?
2. How do you enjoy being touched? Gently caressed? Do you like being spanked hard?
3. Do you enjoy ointments, essential oils, creams etc. on your body? Do these applying these bring you arousal?
4. Do you like coolness or heat? Would you want an ice cube pressed against your body? Would you want to engage in sexual activity by a fire?

Now, reflect and observe what smells are to your liking:

1. Do you have a particular fragrance you enjoy?
2. What smells are welcoming to you? The smell of pine or oak? The fresh air of the mountains?
3. Do you enjoy the smell of food or a drink? Do these smells arouse you?

Finally, do not underestimate the power of taste in sexual activity:

1. Do you enjoy tasting your partner? Do you like having any part of their body in your mouth?
2. Would you eat or lick any edible off your partners' body?

The above is quite a handful! You do not have to find the answers to all the questions immediately. Nor do you have to have anything set in stone. You and your partner should take the time to determine what you enjoy the most from the realm of the visual, the aural, the physical, the smells, and the taste!

Well, that is it for this chapter! If you continue to practice these exercises, it will help you prepare yourself for the experience of Tantric Sex. Now, it is time to introduce Tantric Sex to your partner. Before you do, it is strongly suggested that your partner reads this chapter as well so you both are on the same page!

It is also important to understand that these tips, techniques and ideas are all used to create a stronger physical and emotional connection between you and your partner.

Chapter Summary

- You must learn about yourself before embarking on this journey with your partner.
- Try the practices mentioned regularly to prepare yourself for Tantric Sex.
- Be aware of the senses and what your sexual preferences are.

In the next chapter, you will learn practices for you and your partner to try.

Chapter Two: Setting The Scene

In this chapter, you will learn how to prepare and awaken the sexual energy with you and your partner.

Now that you have accustomed yourself to the practices to prepare you for Tantric Sex, it is time to open up to your partner.

The best way is to share what you have learned is through your exercises with your partner. And no, this does not mean hand them your notebook and ask for feedback! You must verbally communicate how the exercises have helped you and how they have turned you on to the idea of Tantric Sex. Your openness and enthusiasm should spark an interest in your partner for Tantric Sex. Have your partner try out the exercises outlined in the previous chapter. Once your partner has become comfortable with the exercises, you should aim to do these exercises together.

Once your partner has become comfortable and has opened up to the idea of Tantric Sex – it is now time for you both to engage in Tantric Sex practices. The first step is to prepare the environment and atmosphere.

Relax!

Before moving on to more sexual practices, it is essential that you and your partner open yourselves up by warming up! As Tantric Sex is about being relaxed in order to open yourself up to experimentation. Here are some great exercises to warm yourself up and relax your mind and body:

1. I am willing to bet you have had a hectic day or have a busy and stressful life in general! This affects our sex lives

tremendously. Ensure that you and your partner destress before moving on. Get rid of any negative emotions you may have; set aside any chores or 'to-do's' that are cluttering your mind. Have a calm mind. For your relaxed body, ensure that you are properly hydrated and that you have eaten properly and rested your body as it needs to be.

2. To remove any possible stresses, here are a few solutions: punch a pillow, clean any clutter, jump around, scream out your frustrations, or shake your body!

3. Ensure that you and your partner take your hygiene seriously. Have a shower or bath beforehand. Do any necessary ablutions such as brushing your teeth or using the bathroom. You should be cleansed and feeling fresh before engaging in any of these practices.

4. Dress the part! While you may be tempted to strip entirely, these first exercises are just to make you and your partner be relaxed. Wear relaxed clothing that does not feel like a burden on your body.

Warm Up

Once you and your partner have relaxed yourselves it is now time to warm each other up for the sexual practices to come! Here are some warm up practices, Tantra style:

1. You and your partner should stand across from one another. You both should be looking at each other intently. Remember the focus you observed earlier. As you look at your partner, be conscious of the features they possess which you find attractive.

2. You and your partner should extend your arms and embrace tightly. Your arms should be around your partners' waist and their arms should also be around

your waist. Ensure that your chests are pressed against each other and that you continue to look at one another intently.

3. As you hug, ensure that you and your partner have your feet firmly planted on the ground. Imagine that you are both 'one with the Earth', and that you are rooted to the ground you stand on, as a tree would be.

You can also practice the above exercise individually. Instead of embracing in unison, you can take turns embracing each other. Remember that there are no rules and you are open to experimenting and deciding what works best for you and your partner.

Next, it is time to shake things up! Hold your partner and shake their body one part at a time:

1. Wrap your hands around each of your partners' arms and shake it until they feel loose in their arms.
2. Hold your partners hands in your hands and shake them until they feel light.
3. Place your hands underneath the breasts (or nipples) of your partner and bounce them with your hands until they feel relaxed.
4. Caress and hold your partners buttocks and shake and bounce them until they feel relaxed.

Once you are both relaxed, it is time to ease the tension even more through massaging. Do this exercise to each other, taking turns with one person giving and the other receiving. While you conduct this massage, observe what makes you and your partner comfortable and relaxed. Tantric Sex is about communicating effectively with one another to understand what will bring the most sexual gratification. Here is what to do next:

1. Stand behind your partner as they bend over; massage their neck, moving down to their shoulders and finally their spine, back and inner legs.

185

2. When this is complete, have your partner lean their body against you and repeat the massage from the previous step.
3. Have your partner follow the above steps on you.

For the final exercise, stand with your legs stretched apart and face each other. Once again focus on your partner and look at them intently. This final exercise should be done simultaneously.

1. Breathe deeply and let your breath out in loud bursts.
2. Keep your tongue on the roof of your mouth and breathe deeply and gently let your breath out.

You can add any other exercises you and your partner wish to do. At the end of this ritual, you and your partner should feel relaxed and have peace of mind; once you are both relaxed you will be able to open up to one another and explore your sexual desires. You will now be prepared for the exciting exercises to come!

Set The Scene

Think about what would arouse you and your partner. The environment should represent that. If you both like a particular fragrance, it should be prevalent throughout the bedroom. Do you both like silence, save for the sounds you both will produce? Or should the ambience contain slow and seductive music by your favorite singers? Tantric Sex also allows for exploring options that complement sexual intercourse. What activities do you have planned to enhance the sexual experience? Here are a few that may spice things up:

A massage is always welcome in Tantric Sex. You are welcome to practice these massage techniques on yourself first before moving on to massaging your partner. Find you and your partners' comfort zone in massaging. The following exercises can be done on yourself as well as on your partner.

1. Apply pressure on the arm until pain is felt. This will determine what the threshold and the comfort zone is. When massaging, you want to ensure you do not apply the pressure which will cause pain – be aware of the pressure you are applying from when you start to when the pain is felt.
2. Practice your hugging! Do you and your partner like a tight bear-hug? A gentle embrace? Find the hugging style that makes you comfortable and adds to your sexual gratification.
3. Find a nice lotion, oil or cream which feels good on the skin for massaging.
4. Find the part of the body which arouses you/your partner when massaged: whether it is legs, breasts, buttocks, etc.

Next, think about your dressing sense. Yes, the fun part of sexual activity is to dress before you undress. Think about what makes you and your partner feel sexy. What clothing makes you feel fun, flirtatious and confident about your body. It can be lingerie or a full costume. Take the time to prepare how you look to arouse your partner. Remember, Tantric Sex is an experience not a quick act, so even outfits that can involve a bit of role playing are welcome! One person can be a police officer, and another can be a thief! The sky is the limit!

Giving And Receiving

By now, you are sure to recognize a pattern in Tantric Sex! It is a fun and playful experience. And what better way to bring fun and playfulness to your sex life than to use some toys. In Tantric Sex, toys can range from something as gentle as a whipped cream to lick off your partners body to a whip for flagellation. As Tantric Sex is open, you do not need to necessarily use a sex toy as a toy. An everyday object can also be used as a sex toy. Be creative but be responsible: not everything can and should be used as a sex toy as it can cause great harm. Experiment, but with precaution!

Once you have set things up, it is time to prepare yourself and your partner. Normally this would be referred to as foreplay but in Tantric Sex it is all part of one sexual experience. There is no difference between foreplay and sexual intercourse – all is essential to the full Tantric Sexual experience! Here is a great ritual to follow which incorporates some of the practices which you have already learned:

1. Embrace one another in the manner that you both have found comfortable and best for sexual arousal.
2. Practice your breathing exercises together. While in your embrace, inhale and exhale intensely. Then move on to inhaling and letting your breath go in loud and exuberant bursts of laughter. Then move on to breathing in deeply and moaning loudly and frequently!
3. As you are now acquainted with the areas of your partners body that arouses them, massage those areas while you are in your embrace.

Another popular form of touch within Tantric Sex is 'giving and receiving'. This has three stages. Before beginning this activity, you and your partner should strip; to make things more exciting, you can always strip each other!

Once stripped, sit across from each other, cross-legged:

1. Have your partner focus their attention on you. Your partners' arms should be rested on his/her legs with palms facing upward. Stroke their head gently and move down slowly to their neck, to their shoulders, to their arms, and finally to their hands. The rule is that they should not touch you in response – to build up the sexual energy within.
2. Give your partner a minute to relax once this activity has been completed. Now run your finger from their forehead (their third eye) to their nose. Caress their lips with your

finger; Move down further and caress their chest and the nipples, and finally stroke their inner and outer thighs. Again, your partner should not touch you in return to awaken and build up their sexual energy.

3. Your partner should repeat the above steps on you now. Remember to breathe and be conscious of your breathing while doing this. As you should be unabashed now, do not worry about laughing or feeling silly while doing this activity. This carefree attitude is welcome and healthy in Tantric Sex!

One pattern you would have noticed by now is that Tantric Sex wants you to awaken your senses in order to enhance the sexual experience. Here are some exciting activities to help you and your partner activate your senses:

1. What *tastes* arouse you and your partner? Do you enjoy licking whipped cream off one another? Do you enjoy consuming fruit during sexual activity? Are there any edibles which are off-limits?

2. An essential aspect of preparing your environment, is *smell*. As I have mentioned before, maybe you can spray the room or rooms with a fragrance you and your partner enjoy. Fragrances or oils or anything emitting a welcoming smell can also be placed on you and your partners body.

3. How can you arouse your partner through *touch* by using an external implement? This goes back to using props which you and your partner enjoy. Think about other things you can use. For example, you may wish to try the giving and receiving activity from above using a feather or a silk scarf to stroke and caress your partners' body.

4. Finally, do not forget the *sound* needed for the ambience. Apart from music, what other sounds can be added to the

ambience to arouse you and your partner? In addition to moaning which has been strongly advocated, are there other sounds which bring arousal: gasping, panting? Are there particular words when whispered into your partners ear will awaken their sexual desire?

Take the time to experiment and try different tastes, smells, touches, or sounds to enhance the sexual experience for you and your partner. This is what makes Tantric Sex fun!

Once you have determined what you and your partners' likes and dislikes are in regard to the senses, here is a fun activity for you both to practice which utilizes these senses:

1. Be seated across from each other as you were in the giving and receiving exercise. As with the giving and receiving exercise, your partner will be seated while you perform the activities. Afterward, your partner can perform the activities on you.
2. Feed your partner with the edibles they enjoy. Take your time in feeding them. For instance, if you want to feed them a cherry or a grape you can caress your partners' lips with the fruit. To prepare for oral practices, you can have your partner lick and suck the fruit before consuming it whole.
3. Tease your partner with smells. For example, see if you can apply a fragrance to the space between their upper lip and nose. Do this in a small dose. If the smell is something which you can hold in your palm, hold it and hold it toward your partners' nose but not directly underneath their nostrils; again, tease them with the smell.
4. For sound, play music softly but audible enough to get your partner in the mood. As your partner enjoys the music (or noise) whisper the seductive words you know they will like gently into their ear.

5. From the previous giving and receiving exercise, you should have determined what are the spots on your partners body where they enjoy being touched the most. Gently caress them in those areas.

Once this is complete, your partner can perform the activity on you.

Before moving on to the next section, speak to your partner on how you felt about these activities. What did you like or dislike about them? What other experiments would like to conduct? How would you like to alter these activities? Are there additional props you wish to use? Are there additional foods, smells, and sounds you wish to add to the environment?

These activities, if practiced, will open you and your partner up and make you understand the benefit of Tantric Sex. By practicing these activities, you will have not only enhanced your sexual life but also have understood more about your partner and conversely, your partner will know more about you. Practice these activities with your partner every now and then; as these activities can be continuously updated and you both can experiment and alter the activities to your liking, you will continue to enhance your sexual experience. These activities will prepare you for the next activities and make you feel more confident and open-minded when you approach a new sexual practice.

By now you should also be practicing the activities learned in the first chapter with your partner. Continue to observe and track your reflections of these activities to explore how you and your partner have developed. This will provide you with inspiration to continue your journey and try new avenues to enhance your sex life in the Tantric style!

Chapter Summary

- Massage is crucial for becoming comfortable for Tantric Sex.
- Set the scene and create an atmosphere which you and your partner will enjoy.
- Continue to experiment as you both explore yourselves with Tantric Sex.

In the next chapter, you will learn Tantric practices specifically for the genitals.

Chapter Three: Genital Practices

In this chapter, you will learn Tantric practices specifically for the vulva and penis.

At the core of sexual activity of course, are the use of genitals. Now that you and your partner have prepared yourselves for Tantric Sex, you will now learn about how to awaken the pleasure in yourself and your partner by focusing solely on the genitals. This chapter will cover techniques for both the penis and the vulva.

Vulva

We will begin with the vulva. If this is the genital that your partner has, you perform the following activities on them; if you are the one with the vulva, your partner can do this on you and you can also perform these activities on yourself!

Make sure the environment is welcoming for anyone who will be engaged in the activity. Once this is complete, the individual with the vagina should lie on their back, naked on a comfortable surface such as a bed. Make sure any requests, suggestions, or concerns are communicated clearly beforehand. Once all is settled, we can begin with massaging. The massage can be done with hands or with something soft like a silk scarf. Here are the steps to take:

1. The hands should be placed, palms down on the vulva, press (to the level of comfort) down on the vulva. Keep the hands pressed down on the vulva and continue to rotate around the vulva to stimulate the pleasure.

2. Find a lubricant, oil, or cream that you or your partner is comfortable with and is safe. This moisture should be applied in gentle doses on the fingers; once this has been done, the giver should gently and slowly stroke the vulva.
3. Repeat the previous two steps, however now you will move from the vulva to the labia. Press the labia (to the level of comfort) and rotate around to stimulate the pleasure. Then proceed to stroke the labia as you did the vulva.
4. Rub your palms together until you feel heat between them and you experience the tingly sensation on them. Once this has been achieved, press the labia together so they touch each other; ensure you are doing this to the level of comfort and hold the labia together to enhance pleasure.
5. Using your thumbs, massage the top of the inner and outer thighs, right underneath the waist. Do this for a couple of minutes to give the labia rest from the previous exercise.
6. As you had pressed the labia together, gently place your hands on the outer labia and gingerly spread it outward. Gently and slowly, blow air on the labia and the clitoris.
7. Gently touch the clitoris. As you touch gently, move your finger away and then touch the clitoris again.
8. Place your thumb on the clitoris and rotate clockwise and then counter-clockwise.

Take a breather and rest before moving on to the next portion. We will now move on to massaging on the inside. Ensure that the fingers of the massager are well-lubricated and are clean. As always, take precautions and ensure that levels of comfort are not broken.

1. Slowly and gently enter the vagina with one or two fingers. If more fingers are desired, you may insert them ensuring the comfort level does not get broken.

2. After entering the vagina, rotate the fingers to the right and press on the right side; then do the same with the left side.
3. Move your finger upward to reach the urethral sponge, above the vagina. Massage as you were before but be gentle and slow.
4. When on the urethral sponge, press gently and pull away. Repeat this motion.
5. Remaining on the urethral sponge, rotate your fingers.
6. As you are doing these exercises, you can also press on the vulva as you were doing before with your other hand.
7. After the receiver has awakened and is feeling aroused, stop and breathe heavily together.
8. Kissing and breathing into each other's neck increases the sexual tension even more.

These above activities can also be done with the use of a vibrator. Ensure that when these activities are being performed that you and your partner communicate; you want to ensure the most comfortable and most pleasurable experience for the both of you. When all these activities, are complete lie next to one another. This point is not for touching or further activity; lie together in your silence and breathe deeply as you did in your initial breathing exercises. You should both feel awakened sexually; these exercises, like the exercises you have learned before is for opening up and exploring your sexuality and your sexual preferences and desires.

Penis

We will now move on to sexual exercises for the penis. Just as with the vulva, the massaging and handling of the penis is to awaken the senses and arouse stimulation. The final goal is not ejaculation (but do not fret if it happens!) but to heighten the mood.

Once again, ensure the environment is welcoming for you and your partner. The following exercises for the penis can be conducted by your partner, or if applicable you may do this on yourself. Ensure that there is sufficient communication between you and your partner. Tantric Sex is about opening up and understanding one another after all.

The receiver should lie on his back in the nude. As the massages and practices on the penis take place, remember that both the giver and receiver should not feel embarrassed to breathe loudly, moan, or laugh. So, let us begin!

1. The penis should be gently stroked; this can be done with the fingers or with a soft implement such as a silk scarf.
2. Rub the penis gently using an ointment of your partners' choice from an oil or a cream.
3. Grab the pubic hair in handfuls and pull it upward in slow, measured movements.
4. Ensuring that you do not breach the level of comfort, you can apply pressure on the penis by squeezing it.
5. Holding the penis from the tip, stretch it to as much as it can go.
6. Conversely, pull the skin downward as much as it can go (be gentle).
7. Place the penis on the belly, press it down and rotate it – first clockwise and afterward, counter-clockwise.
8. With a lubricated or oiled hand, rub the penis in different directions to enhance the heat.

Ensure that while these practices occur, both you and your partner are breathing heavily as you have practiced. After these exercises, you and your partner should feel aroused and ready to explore more areas of the Tantric Sexual experience.

Take a moment to relax and reflect on what you and your partner have experienced. You should both have been taken to heights you have not been before. You will have both learned more about each other's' comfort levels and sexual desires. You are now more prepared than ever for further experimentation.

Chapter Summary

- Have an understanding of both the vulva and the penis.
- Follow the different techniques to pleasure the genitals.
- Remember that cumming is not the end goal, it is to build sexual energy.

In the next chapter, you will learn some additional sex positions for you and your partner.

Chapter Four: Additional Positions

In this chapter, you will learn a few additional positions in Tantric Sex.

You and your partner have achieved quite a lot! You have both opened yourself up and explored avenues of Tantric Sex which bring you fulfillment. Tantric Sex, as you have learned, is about experimenting. Here are some sexual positions which you may want to try to continue to explore your sexual desires.

Oral

As far as Tantric Sex is concerned, the G-Spot on a woman is within the vagina. The vagina is believed to hold Kundalini, the primary sexual energy found in women. When oral sex is performed on the woman, attempts should be made to stimulate the G-Spot by focusing on the vagina. Here are some positions and techniques for oral sex on the vagina:

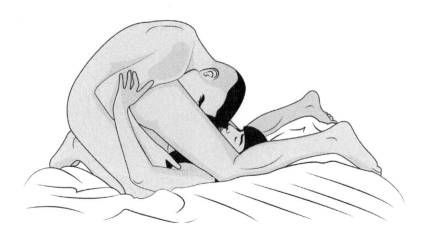

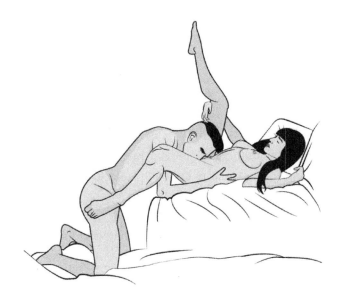

- The tongue should enter the vagina and move around; attempt to touch the roof of the vagina.
- Gently, then rapidly blow air into the vagina.
- Do not forget about kissing! Recall how you learned about spreading and pressing together the labia – both techniques can be done while the labia is kissed.

To continue with kissing, the act of kissing on the lips may seem ordinary but there is a Tantric Sex approach to kissing your partner on the lips.

- With kissing, one person should inhale while the other exhales. This can be switched around afterward; ensure your lips are locked for as long as possible.

For oral sex on a man, the man should have his penis teased. Here is a great technique:

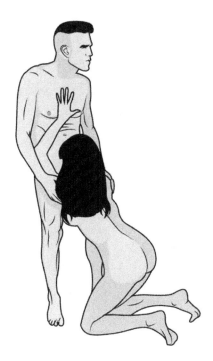

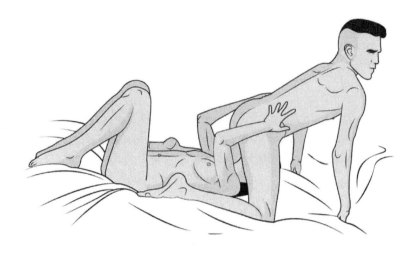

- Kiss the tip of the penis gently, then aggressively. Do it in a 'staccato' movement: kiss quickly, move away and kiss again. Repeat a few times.
- If the receiver is standing while the giver is on their knees it enhances the experience. The receiver can also hold the givers' head.

For pleasuring from oral sex at the same time you can also experiment with the 69 Positions.

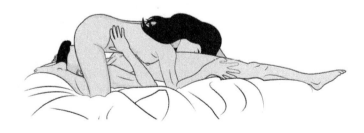

Additional Positions

Here are some more positions to try out:

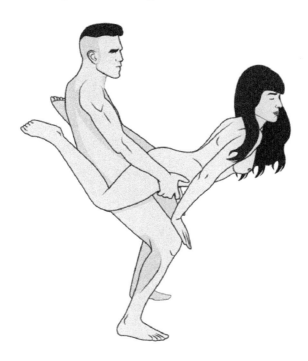

The Mermaid

- The giver can hold the receiver around the waist tightly; the receiver can hold on by using the givers' knees if possible; the giver will penetrate the receiver. If this is too challenging, the receiver can lie down on the bed using it as support.

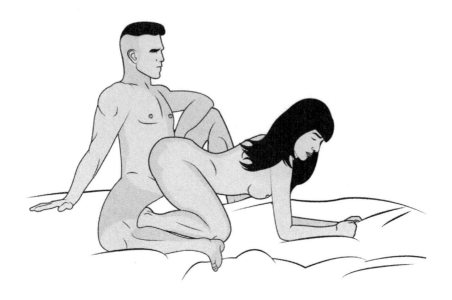

Laidback Larry

- The giver can sit with one leg on the floor and the other raised up; the receiver will have their back arched and will be on all fours with their knees on the bed or floor. The buttocks on the receiver will lay on their back legs while the giver penetrates from behind. The giver can look back her partner while he spanks her and opens up his attraction and love for her.

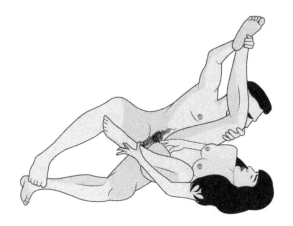

T-Bone

- For this position, the receiver has their legs in the air while the giver lies across and penetrates them; the receiver may caress and massage the givers buttocks. This Position is different and therefor hits a different angle of the vagina leading to increased sexual arousal. Talking to one another in this position is a way to increase the sexual tension also

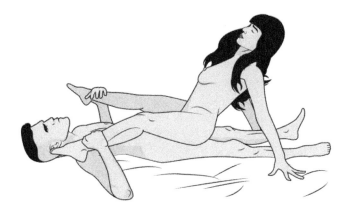

Paddle Boat

- For this position, the receiver has their legs spread as does the giver; the receiver is seated on top. Both partners can clutch at each other's' legs while the receiver is penetrated by the giver. This Position allows the man to rest and puts the woman in full control expressing her love for her partner as she thrusts up and down.

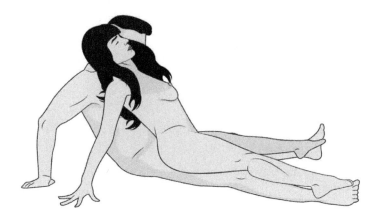

Spin

- The giver uses their hands to support themselves and has their legs stretched out. The receiver sits on the giver and can either be penetrated by the giver or can straddle the giver. The receiver may rest their back on the giver's face; in turn, the giver can kiss or lick the receivers' neck, ears and back.

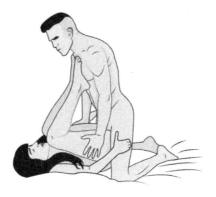

The G-Force

- With this position, the receiver lies on their back with their knees pulled towards their chest. The giver is kneeling and can penetrate the receiver. Placing a pillow under the woman's buttocks allows for an easier angle to penetrate from. Also for harder and stronger thrusts the man can either have one leg up in a lunge position or 2 legs up and feet planted in a squatting position.
- With the position that the receiver is in, the giver can also give the receiver a massage and perform oral sex as well!

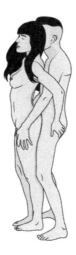

The Wall

- Remember practicing pushing your pelvis forward and your buttocks out? Those practices tie in to this position. The receiver bends forward as much as they can while pushing their buttocks out as much as possible. The giver pushes their pelvis out as much as they can. The giver can penetrate the receiver as well as massage the receiver.

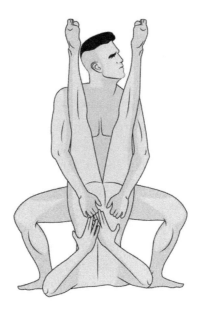

Rabbit Ears

- This exercise is tricky but it's always important to spice up the positions in the bedroom. One person will stand on their head, supported by the other person holding them firmly. The man can enter the vagina on his partner while also massaging or slapping their buttocks.
- An alternative is that the first person can also massage the second person's genitals.

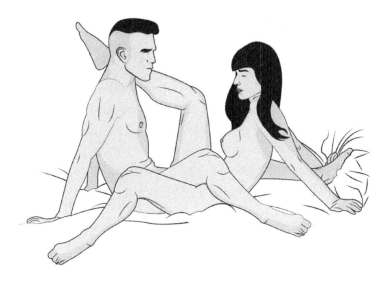

Broken Flute

- Remember one of your first experiences in this book was to sit across from your partner cross-legged? Now that you have gone through that experience, sit across from your partner and intertwine as shown in the image. Penetration is welcome; both individuals should hold each other and caress and massage each other – beginning from the neck, moving to the chest, and working your way downward.
- Slow thrusts while making eye contact enhances the Tantra being formed through one another also

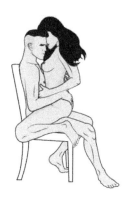

Kneeling Mastery

- In this positions the man will be seated and the woman will sit on top of her partner front on in a cuddling position. This position is a very passionate and loving positions because both partners can make eye contact while they're kissing each other's neck, breathing moaning loudly into each other's ears and telling one another why you love them and what they can do to arouse you even more. If you're both into dirty talk then do that also.

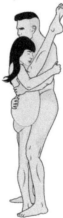

The Ballerina

- This standing sex position can be performed anywhere. The kitchen, the bedroom, the shower. The man will stand erect while the woman lifts one leg up and rests it on her partner's hip as he holds the leg up for her. Both partners can make eye contact while saying what ever they feel comfortable with.

These are the best Tantric Sex practices encouraged. Remember that Tantric Sex is open to interpretation and to experimentation. The exercises you have learned in this chapter and the preceding chapters are intended to open you up to further sexual exploration. It is all about enhancing the physical, emotional and sexual chemistry ach of you have for one another and building on the for the rest of time. You are now well into your Tantric Sex journey, and I encourage you to explore as much on this journey as you can!

Chapter Summary

- The sexual positions in this chapter can be practiced for spicing up your sex life.
- These positions are a foundation; you can continue to experiment in different ways.
- Oral sex is essential to the Tantric Sex experience for both men and women.

Final Words

Do you recall the notebook you and your partner kept at the beginning of your journeys? It is time for you both to bring the notebooks out. Here are some fun final exercises to reflect on your experience with Tantric Sex so far:

1. Swap notebooks with each other and read.
2. After reading, discuss your Progress Logs with each other. Ask each other how you have improved in the four initial exercises.

Return your notebooks to each other and answer these questions:

1. How have you felt over this journey of Tantric Sex?
2. What aspects of your sexuality did you discover? Are there new positions you found that you enjoyed? What about your environment? Did you enjoy which you did not know about before? Focus on the positive aspects, do not waste your time writing about what you did not like or care for.
3. Write about what aspects of the visual you enjoy? What did you learn about yourself in this regard? Repeat for the physical aspect, sounds, smells, and taste.

Every now and then you should reflect upon your observations. It will show you whom you were before you embarked on your Tantric Sex journey and where you are now. Tantra is about discovery and with Tantric Sex you will have learned about you and your partner's sexual desires.

Your sexual energy should now be flowing through your body. Your approach to sex and sexuality has now changed. You will no longer see it as a simple, mechanical act but as a way of life. Tantra is a philosophy that holds to a holistic and connected view of the world; similarly, Tantric Sex should make you realize that you are to use your entire body for sexuality; that having an awareness of the senses should add to your sexual experience; you and your partner will have a more unabashed approach to sexuality and will feel more gratification.

You would have also noticed after applying these teaching that your sexual and emotional connection you have for one another would have highly increased, creating a more loving and exciting relationship for you both.

I want to thank you for reading this book. Remember to refer to this book every now and then to continue on your journey with Tantric Sex. This is a wonderful journey you have embarked upon, and the best thing about it is that there is no destination – Tantric Sex is a continuous journey of discovery, experimentation, and most importantly: bliss.

If you enjoyed the information and teachings in this book please take the time to leave me a review on Amazon. I appreciate your honest feedback, and it really helps me to continue producing high quality books.

Printed in Great
Britain
by Amazon